THE
WHOLE
TOOTH

THE
WHOLE
TOOTH

Stories from The Singing Dentist
guaranteed to make your smile *better*

DR MILAD SHADROOH

First published in the UK in 2023 by Short Books,
an imprint of Octopus Publishing Group Ltd
Carmelite House, 50 Victoria Embankment
London, EC4Y 0DZ

www.octopusbooks.co.uk

An Hachette UK Company
www.hachette.co.uk

10 9 8 7 6 5 4 3 2 1

A CIP catalogue record for this book is available from the British Library.
ISBN 978-1-78072-4720

Printed and bound in Great Britain by Clays Ltd, Elcograf S.p.A

This FSC® label means that materials used for the
product have been responsibly sourced

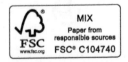

CONTENTS

FOREWORD

Dentistry has always been a rather stoic profession. Dentists have traditionally been seen as the harbingers of doom, without humour or compassion. The phrase 'I hate going to the dentist' is almost as common as 'it's coming home' during a World Cup.

But once in a while, in every million people, you get a singularity. Someone who sees the world in a totally different way. Someone who has the charisma and intelligence to work it to their advantage. Let me introduce you to 'The Singing Dentist', also known as Milad Shadrooh.

My first memory of Milad was at Bart's and The London School of Medicine and Dentistry. It was freshers' week and there was a blind date competition going on. Some plonker had decided to dress up as Ali G and was acting just like him. He was, in fact, pretty amazing and made all the other contestants pale into insignificance. In that moment I thought, 'This guy is wasted on teeth; he is destined for something much bigger.'

Fast forward five years and this same joker has qualified, and is a highly skilled dentist. Milad and I were in different social circles at dental school, but after a couple of chance meetings we really started to get along. From a few trips to Malta, dental award ceremonies, a Gumball car rally, and some crazy crazy nights with him acting as my go-to wingman, we have had some fantastic adventures together. I am proud to call him my best friend.

Not many people will know, but Milad actually had an impressive music career before the birth of The Singing Dentist. He was a signed recording artist during dental school and even went on tour! He has also played sets and been a regular DJ for clubs in London and across Europe.

It's such an amazing journey and something that no other dentist in the history of the UK (and perhaps the world) has managed to achieve. He has made the general public start to love, laugh with and take notice of their dentist. His parodies, mixed with important oral health advice, have taken over social media. His

Ed Sheeran cover has had over 100 million views on different social platforms and was even noticed by the main man himself.

Not being one to rest on his laurels, Milad has been regularly reinventing himself. Projects have included his own calendar, toothpaste and children's comics, not to mention the almost weekly appearances on TV and radio. He has become THE dental social media influencer.

The real question is where he goes from here. Only time will tell!

Nilesh R. Parmar

PREFACE

O ne day at work, a patient cancelled on me. They were due to have root canal treatment, so a 45-minute slot had become open. Unexpected breaks in a list of back-to-back appointments are always welcome. I set about writing up some notes, preparing for the next patient, when 'Hotline Bling' by Drake came on the radio. Tune. I had been practising as a dentist by now for several years, but I had never quite given up on my first love, music. I'd kept up with old rapper and DJ friends, taken time out for music tours and even been approached with a record deal.

And so there I was rapping along when my lightbulb moment arrived.

'You used to call me on my cellphone.'

'I should have never done that endo' (in reference to

'endodontics', which is basically another term for root canal treatment).

Hahaha. A parody freestyle about the risks of root canal treatment and how patients hate it. Why not? I thought it'd be jokes. I had my starting point and quickly penned the rest of the lyrics. Then I got my phone out, opened YouTube and played the Drake track again.

Filming myself, I rapped along with my new lyrics, eyebrows popping all over the place as I settled into the music.

I should have never done that endo
Especially with those curvy roots
Shouldn't have done that endo
Should have just pulled out that tooth
'Cause when I felt that canal twist
I knew my file would break to bits
And when I saw the apex missed
Should have sent him to a specialist
I should have never done that endo
Especially with those curvy roots
Shouldn't have done that endo
Should have just pulled out that tooth
Now what am I gonna do?

I'm sitting here I'm feeling blue
'Cause I know my notes are poo
All this headache for a band 2
I should have never done that endo . . .

Hahaha. My first parody. That evening I sent it to a mate of mine who's also a dentist, Dr Payman. Minutes later he sent a text back.

Dr Payman: Bruv, this is so funny. How did you come up with those lyrics?

Milad: Well, it's just freestyle, isn't it?

Dr Payman: Bro, you should put this online. It'll go viral!

Milad: What you on about? It's stupid, just a laugh. My eyebrows look stupid and people won't know what I'm on about. And dentists don't do this kind of stuff.

Dr Payman: I don't care, I'm going to post it.

Milad: Don't post it, man, please. It's embarrassing.

If only he had listened to me. If he hadn't posted that video, then none of this would have happened to me. I would have stayed Dr Milad, happily freestyling dental parodies to my mates and my mates only.

After our brief exchange I jumped in the shower and left my phone on the side. As I lathered up, I could see my phone going nuts. It kept lighting up, vibrating and ringing with all sorts of notifications.

What the hell was this?

I washed off, dried myself and then checked to see what the fuss was about. Dr Payman had posted the video. He'd posted it, and people had liked it. Not just liked it. Loved it. They were messaging me to say how funny it was. And yet Dr Payman hadn't even posted it into the public sphere. He'd only uploaded it to a closed dental group.

Then, before I knew it, the video had been shared by members of the group into the public sphere. A well-known dentist stumbled upon it and shared it with his sizeable following. All the time, my phone was hotter than an autoclave (the machine we dentists use to pressure-cook our instruments to sterilise them).

In the first three days, the video was viewed more than 300,000 times.

Bloody hell.

That's mad.

What had I done?

1

WHY WOULD ANYONE WANT TO BECOME A DENTIST?

'No offence, mate, but I hate you lot!'

Imagine hearing that every day when you're at work.

To be fair, it's usually followed up by 'It's not you that I hate. It's just . . . why would anyone want to do your job?'

Why *would* anyone want to do my job?

Well, let's answer that question. To do so, we need to go back to Iran in January 1982. There's a cute little chubby baby with big curly locks who's about to celebrate a major milestone. That baby isn't yet known as The Singing Dentist. That'll come later. For now, he's just Milad Shadrooh.

The baby is sitting on the floor of the flat that is his home in the country's capital, Tehran. His dad is in the corner of the room, sitting at the family organ as always. His dad's fingers are on the keys, as if about to pounce into one of the Stevie Wonder numbers or Italian folk ballads he's so fond of. But his dad's eyes are watching the baby's every move. The baby's mum is racing back and forth between the kitchen and the living room, bringing out plates of sweet-smelling Persian food for guests. The aroma of herbs and spices wafts through the room as the baby's grandparents and aunts and uncles tuck in. None of them are looking into the gigantic aquarium full of tropical fish that runs along one side of the room. All of them are watching for what the baby does next. The baby is unfazed by the audience. Around him on the floor are various ornaments and objects, each symbolising a profession. The coloured crayons represent art. The toy scissors mean hairdressing. A piece of wood for carpentry.

Whatever the baby plays with most is what he will be destined for in life. This is all part of the milestone. We call it Gaaz Forooshan. It's a tradition that is popular throughout northern Iran, particularly in Gilan, the region of the country his mother's side of the family is from. The ornaments and objects that surround the baby are only part of the ceremony. He's already completed the other part of it, crawling around from plate to plate and sampling all the wonderful new foods that are perfectly soft for his new tooth. While the audience munched away on chelo kaboob, he sampled the squishiness of banana and the intriguing texture of watermelon.

But now he's eaten, the sizeable audience is keen to see the main attraction. The objects around him have been passed down through the ages, embraced and discarded by the generations that have come before. And now the baby is looking around, wondering what to play with. Where does his future lie? There's a football in the corner. Nope. He doesn't fancy it. There goes any dream of becoming the next Diego Maradona. How about the hammer? It's just lying there, ready to be the first step on a pathway to a life in construction perhaps? Maybe not, the baby doesn't fancy that either, which is a shame because builders are making a fortune in the property game! The baby has just cost himself a hefty chunk of future earnings. Wait. Hold on. What's that?!

The baby stares at it. Ooh, that looks fun. He reaches out and picks it up, then pushes the back of the contraption to squish the air out. And again. He pulls the back out and squishes the air out. And again. And again. Listen to that laughter. He's loving this!

The crowd watch on with interest as the baby carries on playing with a syringe. Tradition and fate have met. It's been decided. The baby is destined to work in the medical profession.

Mic scratch. Freeze frame. Voice over.

It wasn't quite so straightforward, of course. I may have appeared destined for the medical profession

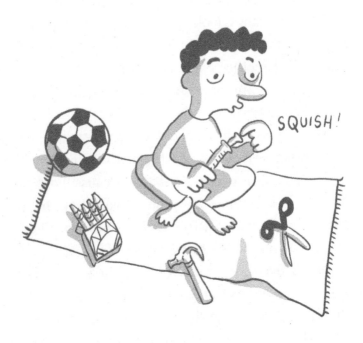

SQUISH!

back then, but fate didn't take into account the other passion that would come into my life: music. Whereas medicine came from the prophecy, music came from my family – in particular, my father. He was an accomplished musician who played the keyboard and was also into production. In our house, music was played the whole time.

In the 1980s, Iran was at war with Iraq, which had terrible consequences, with millions of lives lost. Everyday life still carried on, but with certain adaptations. For a young child like me, the biggest hardship was not having much television to watch. The alternative to TV was bootlegged videos. There was a 'video man' in our neighbourhood who had all sorts of videos in stock, plenty of them from the western world, and plenty from a young singer called Michael Jackson. I used to borrow these videos on repeat and watch them over and over again, transfixed, trying to learn the dance moves and how to moonwalk.

Aside from Persian music, Dad was big into his jazz and soul. Stevie Wonder, Chaka Khan, George Benson, Earth, Wind and Fire, and of course MJ would always be playing in the house.

When I was five, my family moved from Iran to the UK. There was a real family affinity for London. My aunt and uncle both lived there and my mum had visited several times. My dad had even got his business administration degree in the UK. He'd work as a business consultant while Mum would work on her favourite project: me. Some say that her degree in child psychology came particularly in handy for that one.

When we moved to our new country, the music moved with us. The same sounds that filled our house in Iran filled our new place in London. Before I could speak English properly, I knew the lyrics to songs without understanding what they meant. On my first day of primary school, I got sat next to another boy called Miles. He was best friends with another boy called Tom and despite the language barrier, we immediately hit it off and we are still best friends to this day, 35 years later! Miles claims that he taught me how to speak English and he may be right, although I'd say that rap music really shaped my use of the English language. Just as impressionable as the other kids in my new class, I started to rap as well as dance. Learning the lyrics to songs came easily to me. TV also helped mould my personality – *The Fresh Prince of Bel-Air*, in particular, was a big influence on my life, and obviously the theme tune was my starting point. Will Smith was my favourite as his raps were also PG with no cussing. 'Summertime' remains one of my favourite songs to this day. After Will Smith, my rap taste started to become a bit more 'gangsta' as I got into NWA, Snoop Doggy Dogg, Notorious BIG and Bone Thugs-N-Harmony.

When I was 10 or 11, I started writing my own raps and trying them out on my mates. Then, at secondary school, came my big chance. There was a school talent show and anyone was allowed to enter. I convinced my mates, Luis and Joe, to join me on stage and perform 'Informer' by Snow, accompanied by my other mates Dita and Pierre on beatbox!

We absolutely smashed it.

My voice hadn't even broken by this point. I was a little Year 7, performing a pop-ragga track to kids twice my size. But as I looked out from the stage to the audience and saw them going nuts, I realised that music was what I wanted to do for ever.

Writing lyrics turned into performing at house parties, which then became 'emceeing' at under-18 events. Drum 'n' bass and jungle music were growing in popularity, and when jungle morphed into garage, I morphed with it, wangling myself onto digital and pirate radio in South London.

But then reality hit. Music was still my dream, but

things were also starting to get serious with my schoolwork and I needed to choose which A-levels to study. These weren't the days when you could just upload a video to YouTube and be discovered by Usher and become Justin Bieber. Social media didn't even exist back then! Nor were there any talent shows on television. If there were, I'd have auditioned for *Britain's Got Talent* and rapped my socks off. I'd have put all my demos on YouTube. But there weren't. At that time, the best way to get discovered was to make a load of songs and then stand outside various record companies' offices and grab one of the Artists and Repertoire (A&R) people in the hope they'd listen. There are even stories of budding musicians posting their songs to A&R people's houses.

Throughout my music experiences, I could always rely on my dad's advice. He'd sampled the industry back in Iran when he'd performed in a band. He'd seen first-hand just how hard it was to break into the industry properly and make a good career out of music. 'You've got this amazing talent,' he would tell me, 'but keep it as a hobby at the moment. The music industry is so unstable. The only way to make it is through a lucky break, and even then, nothing is guaranteed. It takes luck to get there, but talent to stay there. Trying to make music your career will give you lots of tough times. You're intelligent enough to become a dentist or a doctor. Follow a vocational pathway where you can have a great lifestyle for your whole career. At the very least, get your degree, then if at that point you want to give music a go you can because you've always got your qualification to go back to.'

It was difficult to hear that from the person I respected most. All I wanted to do was music, but I didn't have the self-belief to go against my dad.

Fortunately, I knew what I wanted to study. I'd known ever since that ceremony when I was just a baby. That's right. If I couldn't pursue music as a career, I was going to be a doctor.

What an immensely important decision to have to make at such a young age! Before that, the toughest decision had always been how to style my hair (ponytail and an undercut, since you ask). Now, at 16, I had to decide the subjects that would define the rest of my life. So, I ticked the boxes for chemistry, maths and physics.

It had to be the right decision. My parents had guided me along that path ever since I had picked up and played with that syringe. However, to be absolutely certain, my school careers adviser recommended I do some work experience. That way I could be sure that life as a doctor was right for me. And it'd look pretty good on my university application form.

I got in contact with a family friend, Fadi, who was training to be a maxillofacial surgeon. Now these guys have done it all. Maxillofacial surgeons – or max fac, as we call them – deal with problems in everything from the neck up. Common issues include cancer, reconstructive surgery and trauma. That means they are doubly qualified: not only do they have to complete a degree in medicine. They also have to do one in dentistry. It's an incredibly difficult speciality to master and one that takes a great deal of time. Typically, max fac surgeons spend five years studying medicine and then do four years at dental school. That's a total of nine years – and even then, there are another three years of hospital rounds to be done before they can get on to a specialist list. So, it's more like 12 years. Plenty do it the other way round and study at dental school first, and then when they graduate and start working, realise they like max fac and go back to medical school to get the qualification. It's a tough slog!

Fadi was due to be on holiday when I needed to do

work experience, but he arranged for me to spend the week shadowing his colleague down at Poole hospital in Dorset. Then, he said the words that would influence the rest of my life: 'Dude, don't just think about working in a hospital. There's also dentistry which is quite different. You should 100% sample both. That way you'll get an insight into what hospital life is like compared to a dental clinic setting.'

OK.

I rang around all the dental clinics close to my family home in Putney. My regular clinic told me that they'd be happy for me to come and complete a week of work experience.

Fadi's words chimed with me. It seemed the perfect mix. An excellent opportunity to get a taste of both fields.

After the first day of shadowing at the hospital, I was absolutely certain, that I *did not want to be a doctor!*

Being on-call in a hospital was like torture for me. You come out of one emergency surgery, have a 20-minute nap, then another emergency surgery patient comes in. Sleep deprivation plus stitching someone's face back on after a road traffic accident did not equal my ideal career.

The next day I watched as two surgeons worked for eight hours to remove a cancerous tongue. The cancer had spread to the jaw and down the lymph nodes and it required careful, focused work. Before my very eyes, the patient's face was completely opened up so that bits could be removed. I was only shadowing, yet I found it incredibly stressful. I didn't want to have to take on such responsibility. It gave me a huge respect for the men and women who have dedicated their lives to this, but there was no way I wanted to be among them.

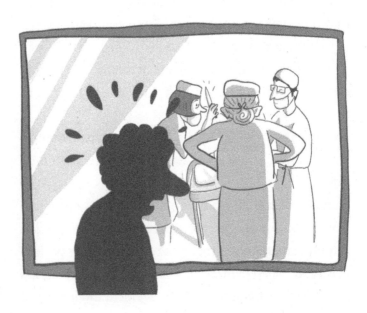

One down, one to go. It felt like the last chance to find the career I had always wanted to follow (except music!). If the dentistry side of things didn't work out, it'd have to be back to Iran to play with those toys again.

The pressure was on. Despite the disappointment that life in a hospital wasn't for me, I had high hopes for dentistry. It ticked all the boxes: a medical profession, science based, plenty of patient interaction, getting to work with your hands and, most importantly for my parents, a respectable job.

From the first moment I stepped into the dental clinic, I got a good vibe. This was more like it. The clinic was on the ground floor of a residential building on Putney High Street. OK, the sea of magnolia that greeted me in reception wasn't beautiful, and the décor was quite bland, but the very fact that a dental clinic could be in a residential building was brilliant. NHS hospitals, more or less, follow the same formula. They look the same, sound the same, smell the same. Yet dental practices can be just about anywhere, from old, listed buildings to portacabins, warehouse blocks and old Victorian houses. This one felt homely. There was none of the high-tech equipment of the hospital, not the white in-your-face rooms. Instead, the reception area felt . . . well, inviting! I had half a mind to pull off my trainers and kick back on one of the sofas with a cuppa!

Before I had the chance, my regular dentist arrived in reception. He greeted me warmly and beckoned for me to follow him into his room. Everything about him was friendly and welcoming, just like the rest of the practice. He was young and bubbly and also Iranian, which helped to break the ice. Most of all, he looked like he was enjoying himself. There was an aura of satisfaction about him, which I found quite inspirational. If a dentist could be that comfortable in his own skin, then maybe I'd found my profession.

The patients trickled in and the dentist made sure to put each of them at ease before starting any procedures. He'd take the time to ask how they were, what they'd been doing and then explain the procedures that were going to take place, working in tandem with the nurse the whole time. Mainly, the procedures were the same: fillings, cleanings, check-ups, extractions. I watched how he used his hands to find solutions to problems. I had often been told I was very good with my hands. I had also been told that I was good at science. These were scientific problems that my family friend was using his hands to solve.

There's no denying that dentistry is a scientific profession.

Between each patient, while the nurse wrote up the notes, he spent time explaining to me what had just happened, what was coming up next and what a day in the life of a dentist usually consisted of. Mainly, he emphasised the importance of patient interaction. 'If you're an amazing dentist but a terrible communicator, patients won't keep coming back,' he told me.

Everything he said was music to my ears. Interacting with people was always something I'd been good at and helping people by interacting with them was exactly what I wanted to do. The importance of working with a small regular group of people fulfilled my desire for teamwork. The business element chimed with me too. You had to provide a good service to keep demand high. Because of my dad's influence, I'd always liked the business aspect of things and the thought of being a business owner appealed. Over those first few days, the dentist told me how dentistry provides loads of options for business, such as expanding your practice, opening up new ones, rebranding and so on. You don't really get that working in a hospital setting.

The dental room, I found, was like an office – well,

an office where the work is done in people's mouths rather than on desks. You arrive every day at 9am and leave every day at 5pm, then come back the next day. There were no late walk-ins or sleep-deprived nights. The surgery doors simply closed at the same time each day and everyone went home to their nearest and dearest. I liked that routine. As in any office, it was the people who made the work environment what it was. First of all, there was the dentist, who gave me plenty of time and made sure that I had a laugh with him between appointments. But then there were also the receptionists, the technicians, the nurse and the patients themselves.

The work itself was a little monotonous but I didn't mind that. After the previous week of seeing faces reconstructed and cancerous tongues removed, monotonous was good. After my third day of shadowing, the dentist turned to me and said, 'Dude, you've pretty much seen everything there is to see now. If you don't want to come for the rest of the week you don't have to. Tomorrow we've got the same procedures as the last few days. It'll be the same the next day, too.'

I'd already seen enough to make my decision.

I was to be a dentist.

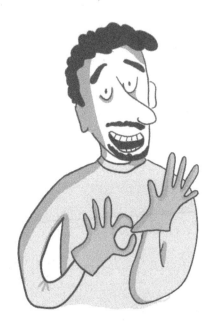

2

A BRIEF HISTORY OF DENTISTRY

Get this: dentistry was going on as far back as 7000 BC. Researchers know this because they found dental drills made of flint that were used all that time ago in the Indus Valley Civilisation. Or, as it's known now, Pakistan.

That discovery makes dentistry one of the oldest medical professions.

The next big milestone came in 5000 BC, when the first known reference to tooth decay was made. Not to worry. The dentists back then were sure they knew what was causing the decay: tooth worms! Those pesky little critters, so small that they couldn't be seen with the naked eye, were burrowing into people's mouths and causing havoc. They'd squirm around the gums and find their way into teeth by digging a hole into them. Once there, they'd wriggle about and cause a great deal of pain to the owner of the teeth. When the tooth worm wiggled, the tooth would ache and ache. And when it stopped, the toothache would stop.

It doesn't reflect well on the dental profession that the tooth worm theory wasn't disproved until the 17th century. And until then, treatment of tooth decay was centred around removing the little pests. Some dentists of the time would attempt to lure the worms out with honey. The theory went that the tooth worm would be attracted by the sweet nectar and poke its head out of the tooth. Upon sight of it, the dentist would grab hold of it and fling it into the bin – seamlessly relieving the patient of their toothache. If that didn't work, however, more radical methods were used. Some dentists chanted spells and handed out potions; others used herbal remedies. Saxons placed holly leaves in boiling water and asked the patient to open wide so that the tooth worms could leap from the mouth and into the water. They'd then give the patient a toothpaste of cinnamon bark, honey and pepper. Aztecs encouraged patients to chew hot chillis to relieve the pain, while Egyptians applied a dead mouse to the affected tooth.

Imagine that!

'Hello, Mrs Smith. How are you this morning? So, what can I do for you today? Toothache? Well, sit down in the chair and open wide. You're scared of rodents, you say? Well, don't worry about that, just close your eyes. No, the mouse won't move! Yes, it's free of diseases – what are you implying about my surgery? OK, here we go. I'll just rub it back and forth a few times. There we go. That's the treatment done. Now, if you'll just go and see Hayley on reception, she'll give you a prescription box of a mouse a day. If you run out, feel free to lay your own traps around your house.'

Unsurprisingly, the mouse treatment didn't spread beyond Egypt. One Chinese text, written in 2700 BC,

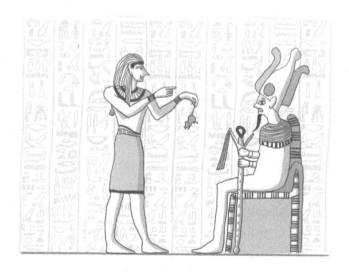

advocated roasting a piece of garlic and 'crushing it between the teeth, mixing it with chopped horseradish seeds or saltpetre, making it into a paste with human milk. Form pills and introduce one into the nostril on the opposite side to where the pain is felt'. I don't know about tooth worms, but that treatment would sure ward off vampires!

The most popular treatment for tooth worms back in ancient times – and even right up to the eighth century in Europe – was removing the nerve of the tooth. After all, the nerve of the tooth is pretty tiny and wiggly, just like a worm. Ancient dentists wouldn't think twice about pulling teeth. Sure, the patient would end up in a lot of pain, but that was only in the short term! Long-term, the treatment proved effective. Without the nerve, the tooth no longer ached. And without the tooth, the pain was never going to come back.

It could be argued that all treatments were effective. A patient would open up their mouth for a dentist to take a look inside and all the dentist needed to do was declare that they couldn't see any tooth worms. Job done! It was better than the mouse technique, at least. . .

The first known dentist was Hesy-Re. Around

A BRIEF HISTORY OF DENTISTRY

2600 BC he worked his magic in ancient Egypt under the modest title of 'Great One of the Dentists'. He also served as a confidant to the pharaoh, but I know which job I'd prefer. And Hesy-Re wasn't the only one at it. Papyrus scrolls from that time confirm that many rich Egyptians employed servants to look after their teeth, in an effort to live their lives in the same way as their great pharaoh. Dentists were considered to be of extremely high status within society. The tricks of their trade included using opium for pain relief. None were rewarded as much as Hesy-Re, however, who was given his own decorated tomb by the pharaoh upon his death with the inscription 'the greatest of those who deal with teeth, and of physicians'.

All the great ancient empires took oral issues seriously. Quite rightly. Greek physicians discovered that teeth are made of bone and contain nerves. They recommended using a dentifrice powder of laurel, cardamom and parsley to rub on teeth and gums to improve oral hygiene. The laurel tree, native to Greece, was considered to have an especially beneficial impact on teeth due to its antiseptic oils and the fresh, healthy scent it left in the mouth.

Today the Hippocratic Oath is still taken by many medics across the UK as a medical school tradition and a means of understanding morals and ethics in the profession. We dentists have our own version:

I will remember that I do not treat a decayed tooth or a cancerous growth, but a sick human being whose illness may affect the person's family and their economic stability. My responsibility includes these related problems, if I am to care adequately for the sick.

That's because back in ancient Greece, the 'father of medicine', Hippocrates, didn't just know a thing or two about medical advances, but also about dentistry. Despite the fact he diagnosed his patients by drinking their urine and having a nibble on their ear wax (if the wax tasted bitter, the patient was healthy; if it was sweet, then they were not), his work was vital in the advancement of dentistry as a science. In their writings, Hippocrates and philosopher and polymath Aristotle gave guidance for stabilising loose teeth with wire, getting rid of teeth with forceps and cauterising of oral tissue, as well as on the development and growth pattern of teeth.

The Romans took the Greeks' discoveries one step further by creating dental crowns and false teeth out of ivory taken from animal teeth, which they'd cut down to size. Tooth size was smaller back then than it is today. Due to their diet of coarse bread which ground teeth down, Romans had short, stubby pegs.

One Roman, in particular, helped develop dental innovations: Celsus. This guy's dental skills were hot. Celsus advised all Romans to wash their mouth out every morning. In a way, he even invented braces. Well, he attempted to align teeth by using the pressure of his fingers, which according to his diaries he managed to do with some success. The Romans really took his advice to heart. They really did wash their mouths out every morning.

With urine.

That's right.

Urine.

These clever Romans, you see, worked out that urine becomes ammonia when it decomposes. Nowadays ammonia is commonly found in cleaning products, and back then they had already realised that ammonia was excellent at removing stains. And so human urine, theirs or their friends', or even animal urine, was gargled and then spat out in an attempt to whiten teeth. It's no surprise that such unique methods created the perfect environment for Pliny the Elder to preach to the converted. In his book, *The Natural History*, Pliny advised those suffering from toothache to go and catch a frog under a full moon and spit into its mouth. Cheaper than a visit to my local dentist, I hear you saying, and you're right. The madness didn't stop there, though. If you didn't also say 'frog, go, and take my toothache with thee!' the cure wouldn't work. Pliny also believed that the ashes from the burnt head of a hare, when combined with nard, made for a great corrective of bad breath.

At least that was preferable to some other dental methods employed by the Romans. It was also believed that the hair of a man who had been crucified, or even the freshly spilt blood of a man violently murdered, could be used to improve oral hygiene.

You might have guessed by now that, even though there had been some bizarre dental practices in centuries past, it was the Romans who were the first to really see the potential in using dentistry for sadistic pleasures. Their idea of using dentistry to inflict pain developed alongside their treatment of toothache. Gone was the garlic. In came the pincers. Dentists agreed with Hippocrates' and Aristotle's writings and decided that extraction was the best possible treatment for toothache. They tended to remove the offending

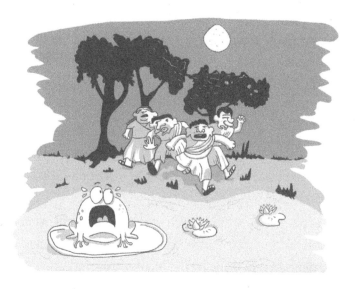

tooth with a set of pincers known as *dentiducum*, or by cutting the gum away from around the tooth and then easing it from its socket. When the authorities got wind of the fact that dentists could inflict pain, they began to use tooth extraction as punishment. Thrown to the lions or sent to the dentist: not much to cheer in ancient Rome!

During the early Middle Ages, monks were put in charge of dental procedures. The reason? They were deemed the most educated citizens, their lifetime of study, sacrifice and piety putting to shame my five years of dental school. But in 1163, when the Church banned them from carrying out procedures, a new solution was needed. Step forward the barbers. They were handy with sharp shaving blades and what else did a dentist need? This, it was reasoned, more than qualified them to extract teeth and perform surgery. Another link to me being destined to be a dentist: I am my own barber and I have the hairstyle of a monk!! Nailed it . . .

In the 12th century, the new dental barbers were considered expensive, though, so many people had their dental work done by the local blacksmith, due to the fact that they owned pliers: how else would one extract a tooth? As time went on, barbers and blacksmiths became responsible for bloodletting to remove pain, carving false teeth from cow bones, extracting teeth and, of course, leeching. But they weren't the only ones who pulled out teeth. As with the Romans all those years before, the powers that be in medieval England recognised how tooth extraction caused pain. Because of this, they regularly used it as a form of punishment. Eating meat during Lent could be punished by the removal of the two front teeth! That's one good reason to turn vegan . . .

As time went on, the dental barbers grew in

confidence and even came up with their own ingenious solutions to oral hygiene. In Tudor times, poo was mixed with honey and then used to remove rotten teeth. If that didn't agree with patients, there was always the option of using boiled frogs. One spoonful of the boiled liquid was considered perfect for soothing toothache. In all likelihood, it probably tasted better than the toothpaste of the time: a mixture of lavender, rosewater and cuttlefish.

The work of dentists got a lot tougher when sugar crept into the population's diet. A trade deal with Morocco proved to be the catalyst, and by the 1590s the British were consuming around 2000 tons of sugar a year. All of a sudden, dentists weren't just dealing with worn teeth, but with teeth blackened by refined sugar.

One of the biggest fans of sugar was the sovereign herself, Queen Elizabeth I. Because of the cost of importing it, sugar came to reflect wealth and status – so much so that people desired black teeth to show that they too were high born. At the royal courts, they wolfed sugar down. Sweets, gingerbread and a 'leach' of milk, sugar and rosewater were all popular with the sweet-toothed Elizabeth. And it wasn't only used in food and drink: Elizabethans believed that sugar had medicinal properties and even used it as a form of toothpaste. Unsurprisingly, Queen Elizabeth's teeth suffered greatly, and a number became decayed – some so badly that she had to have them removed (by now, tooth removal had become normalised). The very first time she was due to have a tooth removed she was so scared that the Bishop of London, who was watching on, offered to have one of his perfectly healthy teeth removed to show that it was a pain-free solution.

That's one way of serving queen and country.

Before the advent of sugar, however, there was another fashion that had caused people's teeth to rot: tobacco smoking. When this was introduced in the 1560s, oral hygiene plummeted. Not that people were aware it was due to tobacco. At the time, it was believed that tobacco had medicinal properties, whereas another new import, potatoes, were viewed with suspicion. A Spanish medic, Nicolas Monardes, wrote a report that recommended tobacco as a medical aid to help cure toothache, worms, lockjaw and even cancer. By the mid 1600s tobacco use was widespread. And after the Great Plague of 1665, it actually became compulsory in establishments as prestigious as Eton College, where its smoke was seen as a defence against 'bad air'. Imagine that – receiving detention for not smoking behind the bike sheds!

It was a strange time to say the least: tobacco was 'healthy' and dentistry could kill you. From the 1600s, the London Bills of Mortality began to list the causes of deaths. 'Teeth' was constantly among the five or six most common causes of death. By the 1660s, 'toothache' was estimated to be the cause of one in ten deaths. How so? You may ask. Well, with every toothache the danger of infection loomed. Without proper treatment, infected abscesses could form between the teeth and gums. These infections could then move into the blood or bone marrow, ultimately causing sepsis. There was also the danger of infection after a tooth extraction, while some poorly performed procedures left the patient bleeding to death. I can see why people back then may have been apprehensive about getting treatment. There are even reports of some people dosing themselves so heavily with opium to relieve the pain that they ended up overdosing.

Something had to be done.

And so there began what we might now recognise as modern dentistry. Exciting new techniques emerged from France, where *dentistes* aimed to provide more preventive and less painful treatment. Extraction was only to be used as a last resort. Dealing with a stylish Parisian elite, the *dentistes* distanced themselves from the butchers who had come before them and attempted to make dentistry a respectable, distinguished profession.

And it worked! Parisians began to visit their dentists not only for pain relief, but also for aesthetic purposes. Good teeth were associated with beauty and wealth. The dentists' success stemmed from methods shared by French surgeon Pierre Fauchard, the 'father of modern dentistry.' In his book *The Surgeon Dentist: A Treatise on Teeth*, published in 1723, he introduced sophisticated ways to remove decay and restore teeth, fill cavities and treat periodontal disease – some of which are still used today. Not satisfied with all that, he was also responsible for, finally, dispelling the tooth worm myth and was the first person to identify the association between sugar and tooth decay. Thanks to his work, dentistry was no longer seen as a lesser form of medicine. What a legend!

French attitudes toward teeth made their way across the Channel. The Age of Enlightenment was getting into full swing, with people all around the world embracing logic, reason and science. Dentistry flourished. Americans started to associate good teeth with success – much to the frustration of George Washington, who was famed for having just one natural tooth left in his mouth by the time of his inauguration as president. Washington had a wide assortment of dentures to cover up his lack of teeth. Some were made of metal, some from the ivory of hippos and elephants, and the rest from the teeth of other people. Disturbingly, records show that he bought some from slaves. After the Battle of Waterloo in 1815, the gruesome practice of making dentures with teeth pulled from the mouths of slain soldiers became popular. With more than 50,000 soldiers killed, 'Waterloo Teeth' dentures flooded the market, bringing the price down so much that it was no longer just the elite who could afford them. They sold like hotcakes at markets and through dental catalogues. With hippo or elephant ivory acting as the gum and the teeth riveted in place with metal pins, the dentures looked OK. But they didn't actually work too well. The gold wire springs used to keep the teeth in the mouth made eating near impossible. Many of the owners of Waterloo Teeth resorted to removing their dentures and having their food mashed or ground down so that they could eat it. Even worse, the gum ivory would soon rot in the mouth – giving off a horrible stench. Ladies took to carrying enormous fans so that they could cover their bad breath.

Back in the UK, the teeth of dead people had long been in demand. In the 18th century, grave robbers used to steal the teeth of corpses, making as much as the equivalent of £10,000 in today's money from a single night's work! Meanwhile, wealthy Georgians wanted fillings made from criminals' teeth. Many even paid for the teeth from poor children, which were yanked from the (still alive) child's mouth and

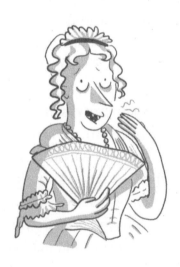

transplanted to their own! This particular trend came about following the publication of failed doctor John Hunter's 1771 book, *Natural History of the Human Teeth*. In his book, Hunter named each of the teeth – names we still use to this day – and drew detailed diagrams. He gave advice on diet and tooth brushing, and particularly on tooth transplants. However, tooth transplants performed according to his instructions rarely managed to take root in the mouth. Worse, they carried the very real danger of passing or spreading infections and diseases such as syphilis. Still, they worked better than the Georgians' fillings, which were largely made of either lead or beeswax. And there was me thinking you should never put anything poisonous in your mouth . . .

Innovations also came in the form of toothbrushes and toothpaste. In 1780, William Addis created the first-ever mass-market toothbrush – from his jail cell! Having been imprisoned for his part in a Spitalfields riot, poor old Addis sat in the corner of his lonely cell, clutching on to the rag that he used to clean his teeth with the latest development in Georgian toothpaste: soot (closely rivalled by brick dust and crushed shell and certainly an improvement on the mixture of urine, sticks and gunpowder that had been popular in earlier times – though initial reports suggested that the mix was quite explosive . . .). Then he saw it: a broom! It was standing there in the corner. Addis looked at the bristles and had an idea. Surely bristles would be much more effective at cleaning one's teeth than a dirty old rag? Addis went on a charm offensive, eventually convincing his prison guard to smuggle him in some bristles. Once that was done, Addis drilled a hole into a bone left over from his supper, tied the bristles through the hole and then sealed them with glue. Eureka! Most people can't wait to get out of prison but following his invention Addis truly was desperate. Soon enough, his wish was granted and straight away he got to work. The toothbrushes he manufactured were expensive – so expensive that those who could afford one would share it with their family – but were quickly lapped up. By the time he died, William Addis was a very rich man. And they say crime doesn't pay!

Things were on the up for dentistry, which was beginning to be widely accepted as a trade and a science. There was still one big problem, though: it hurt. A patient would have alcohol splashed on their face or poured down their throat to try to numb the pain while the dentist removed their teeth. Which you can imagine, was still pretty painful, especially if the procedure involved a cauterisation of the nerve endings using red-hot wire. Step forward Cornish chemist Humphry Davy. In 1799, while a science student at Bristol, Davy found that rather than splashing alcohol on the person's face, getting them to inhale three large doses of nitrous oxide could help relieve pain – and cause laughter.

He shared his findings, and tried – unsuccessfully – to prove the efficacy of nitrous oxide at a public demonstration, but it would take more than half a century for his research to be applied to dentistry. During that time, patients had to grin and bear it with a face full of alcohol while other scientists experimented with anaesthetics. Henry Hickman trialled carbon dioxide. Friedrich Serturner isolated morphine from opium. Then, in 1842, William Clarke and American dentist William Morton proved the benefits of using ether as an anaesthetic. In 1845, they administered ether during a public dental procedure to much greater success than Davy had managed with nitrous oxide 50 years earlier, proving it to be a more potent anaesthetic. Over time, however, nitrous oxide would also come to be accepted as an anaesthetic and it continues to be used in dentistry today. Still, experimentations with other anaesthetics continued: from chloroform to cocaine. Karl Koller, a student in Vienna and classmate of Sigmund Freud, was a particular advocate of cocaine, discovering that injecting it could deaden nerves and block signal-conduction in the ones that caused pain. It could even be used to target individual teeth rather than the whole mouth. And it proved more successful than chloroform, which became associated with fatalities. Sure, chloroform could be effective, but there was little room for manoeuvre in its administration. Just enough could desensitise a patient; too much could paralyse the lungs and result in death.

Opium . . . cocaine . . . the dental practices of the past probably had more in common with a seedy nightclub than the surgeries of today!

While such experimentation was going on, dentists continued to run their surgeries and even advertise their services in local newspapers. Their advertisements weren't always totally accurate – especially because anybody could set up as a dentist. Would-be amateurs soon found out that dentistry wasn't as easy as it looked, however, and with cowboy dentists on the rise, further innovations were required to put patients at ease. A creation by London dentist James Snell, a reclining chair, improved the patient experience.

A clockwork-powered dental drill, created in 1864 by British dentist George Fellows Harrington, significantly speeded up procedures. Though the drill has long been associated with feelings of anxiety and horror (the first drills date back more than 9000 years and were thought to be used to release 'evil spirits'), its development not only enabled dentists to make procedures quicker, but also less painful.

Towards the end of the century, a new landmark was reached when the UK Dental Act was passed in 1878. One year later, the British Dental Association was formed. By this point, cowboy dentists had been legislated out of business, with requirements for all dentists to be on a register held by the General Medical Council.

These were exciting times, as businesses woke up to the commercial opportunities within dentistry. Marketing for various toothpastes and formulas proliferated. Characters were created to encourage children to look after their teeth. In Britain, many European countries and the US, they still have the tooth fairy; in Hispanic countries it's a mouse called El Ratoncito Pérez. France also has a mouse: 'La Petite Souris'. In some Asian countries, children throw a tooth that has fallen out onto the roof and ask for it to be replaced with the tooth of a rodent (though in South Korea they believe that a magpie will find the tooth and bring a gift in return). Rodents' teeth never stop growing – and they definitely exist – so it makes sense to have a tooth mouse rather than a tooth fairy. Especially when not all tooth fairies are nice. In Lancashire, legend had it that Jenny Greenteeth would hang around local ponds and drag children who didn't look after their teeth into the depths of the water. Staying on the evil pathway, Finland has 'Hammaspeikko', the tooth troll. If Finnish children eat too many sweets and don't look after their teeth, they're said to lure the tooth trolls.

These characters weren't necessarily created as educational devices. Myths and legends have existed almost as long as dentistry has, eventually evolving into the characters that we all know and love today. Vikings believed that children's teeth gave them good luck and wore them as a charm when going into battle. Such was the power of this belief that they even paid children for their baby teeth. If I had to choose between selling my tooth to a fairy or a Viking, I know which one I'd go with. In other Norse traditions, children's baby teeth were buried when they fell out to spare them from hardship in the next life, while in the

England of the Middle Ages, they were burnt for the same reason. Failure to do so would mean the child would spend their entire afterlife searching for the tooth. Apparently.

For some reason, in the early 20th century, rather than avoiding tooth extraction at all costs, people started going a bit crazy for it. In 1930s and 40s Britain, aristocrats chose to have all their teeth removed and to wear dentures instead. They considered it the best way to have good-looking teeth while saving themselves from a lifetime of expensive dental treatment. There was also the bonus that dentures would never give them toothache. Tooth removal became the perfect gift for an 18th or 21st birthday, or even as a wedding present.

The creation of the NHS in 1948 changed everything. Suddenly dental treatment became affordable and regular visits to the dentist for check-ups became the norm. People knew that they needed to maintain oral health, and dentists knew they needed to perform preventive as well as reactive dentistry. The work of the *dentistes* all those years previously had shone through. The increasing popularity of the press and television, and in particular the development of the camera, further strengthened the subliminal link between good teeth, beauty and success. You don't think Marilyn Monroe would have been so iconic if her teeth had been the same colour as her hair, do you?

The trend continues today with cosmetic dentistry. Patients no longer visit the dentist solely to prevent problems, but to improve their appearance. Teeth whitening, teeth straightening and smile makeovers are just some of the numerous treatments on offer. Celebrities such as Jimmy Carr 'want it to look like someone's opened a fridge' when they open their mouth. And, as dentists, our job is to help our patients achieve their goals. We always want patients to feel better after treatments, whether that's because their appearance has been improved or their pain has been reduced.

Dentistry has come a long way and it will continue to advance thanks to the skill of those within the profession. I'm sure that future generations will look back at what we are doing now and say, 'I can't believe they actually used drills and gave injections! The barbarians!'

Yet, despite all our advancements, the dental chair is still strongly associated with feelings of fear. All those years of painful pulling, dreadful drilling, diseased dentures and terrifying dental torture have burnt into our collective conscience. We still routinely use phrases like 'pulling teeth' to describe frustration. It seems that, when it comes to dentistry, history has a lot to answer for.

3

HOW TO BECOME A DENTIST

When people ask what I do for a living and I tell them that I'm a dentist, I usually get one of two reactions:

- They hide their teeth because they're embarrassed and afraid that I'll judge them (I don't).
- They say 'Why do you do it? I can't think of anything worse than looking into someone's mouth all day.'

Yep. Dentistry definitely has a stigma attached to it. I'd get less grief if I told people I do colonics all day. Sticking pipes up people's bums, it seems, would be preferable to looking inside their mouths.

For the chance to get such social judgement, you need a list of qualifications longer than a string of floss and a single-minded focus that begins not long after leaving the womb. Before you're legally allowed to vote, join the army or buy a lottery ticket, you need to have chosen dentistry as your future career path.

In the UK, your GCSEs govern your A-levels, which determine your degree, which leads to your profession. Some degree subjects open you up to numerous pathways. Study English and you could end up in careers as diverse as teaching or law. If you want to become an account manager, you can study any one of a number of different degrees. If you want to become a dentist, however, you have to study for a degree in dentistry. A 2:1 in sociology won't convince a dental clinic you're the right person to handle its patients' teeth.

Deciding to study dentistry is therefore a decision that will affect upon the rest of your life. Thousands of bleary-eyed teenagers, tired from spending all night gaming on *Fortnite*, are forced into making this momentous decision at the tender age of 13 when they make their GCSE subject choices, which have to have a focus on the sciences. By the time they've dropped their games consoles in favour of Tik-Toking or Snapchatting in search of romance, they're forced into

A-level choices. And again, all three core sciences are demanded, with top grades in each.

When the decision to study a degree in dentistry is made, you're in it for the long haul! And if you go on to dental school from university, you're going to end up working with teeth. If you want to work with something else, you have to go back to the start and pick another degree. That's the only way. Which is crazy, because most university students can't even decide whether to spend their money on food or alcohol, let alone what they want to do every day for the rest of their life.

It could be said that the decision to become a dentist is reached even earlier than the age of 13. Many people want to become a dentist because someone in their family is a dentist. For some it is an Iranian prophecy. And for others, money is a motivator too. There is no point in denying it. You can love teeth more than anything but it is always nice to be paid well. Dentistry is a well-paid profession.

What is certain is that the decision to become a dentist will be influenced by a person's upbringing. When I started dental school, there were 60 people in my year; 59 of them came from private schools. Just one had studied at a state school and he was super intelligent. There are of course plenty more super intelligent state-school students who'd make fantastic dentists, and it is a shame they're being lost along the way.

Academic diligence is non-negotiable for any would-be dentist. But even this may not be enough to convince the powers that be that a student deserves a place in dental school. That's because dentistry isn't just a science.

There's around one place at dental school for every 10 applicants. Most of those 10 applicants are going to have decent grades. Those with the top grades are going to be the ones who get invited to interviews. This is when the school can do their best to work out which applicants will make the best dentists. What skillset do they have? Are they good with people? Do they seem trustworthy characters?

When I sat on the interview panel for my dental school, I came across many super-intelligent students who would have been great in a dental lab, but not in a dental clinic. They would have been able to speak to bugs, but not to actual people.

So, yes, interpersonal skills are just as important as knowledge in dentistry. You can learn science, but some personality traits are inbuilt. At times it can be a pressurised environment where you need to deliver bad news to a patient. You have to be psychologically fit, compassionate and understanding to do this. Otherwise, the patient will go to a different clinic or, even worse, be put off seeking further treatment.

Manual dexterity is also important. Playing the violin while doing root canal treatment isn't the norm and dentists aren't expected to be able to slam-dunk their old notes into the wastepaper bin. But, weird though it may sound, when applying for dental school, the fact that you play an instrument or have been competing regularly in a sport is a way to show off your manual dexterity and hand–eye coordination. Combined with good grades, it improves your chances of succeeding in the interview.

I loved dental school. Mine was the concisely named Queen Mary and Westfield, St Bartholomew's and The London School of Medicine and Dentistry, when the whole new cohort of students gathered together in a massive auditorium. The dean of the dental school came on stage and welcomed us all. 'I stand here today and look out before me at all the bright young future medical carers of this country.' It was inspirational stuff. It made us feel great to be there.

I'm sure there was a syllabus in those first few

weeks, but in reality, the start of university is all about one thing: freshers. The benefit of the dental school being amalgamated with Queen Mary University of London was that we got to take part in all the activities arranged for students on other courses, too. For the vast majority of us, it was the first taste of freedom, the first time living away from home. And did we make the most of it!

I lived in halls on campus with a friend from school, Luis. Technically, I wasn't supposed to live in halls because I was from London. However, commuting from my home in Putney was an hour and a half one way. Fortunately, Luis had moved to Oxford at 16 and qualified for halls. Even more fortunately, the only halls accomodation that he was offered was a married couple's kind of room with a big double bed and a sink in the corner. The rent was slightly higher than it would have been for a single room so he asked if I could share with him and split the cost. I was keen and so we did (luckily the double bed was made of two singles – problem solved!).

Living with Luis was wicked. He was into music and had lots of DJing equipment in the room. Over the year, we worked up to doing uni club nights together, him DJing and me emceeing. We also spent plenty of time socialising with the others in the halls while we all learnt about living on our own for the first time.

Pejman was the first person I met there on my first day. He seemed more mature than most, which was probably to do with the fact that he had already completed a degree in neuroscience. He was Iranian as well – it's weird how we cluster together. On my other side was Jean-Paul, who was from a family of dentists in Malta. His father and grandfather were dentists, while his sister was in her final year of dental school. Past him was Nilesh, the first Asian guy with an Essex accent I'd ever met! Who knew we would become the best of friends in years to come. Making up the little group was Dipen. While the others talked, he listened. He was short, slight and shy. When you asked him a question, you really had to prick up your ears to hear his response.

Dipen became my work partner, and his transformation over the five years of dental school was one of the highlights of my time there. With the support of those around him, Dipen came out of his shell and emerged as a funny guy with an infectious sense of humour.

It took me far less time to come out of my shell. Within the first few weeks of freshers, I'd made sure that all my fellow students knew me. There was a blind date event with our rival dental school, King's College London. I put myself forward as a participant, but with a twist: I'd take part as Ali G. This was around the time that Sacha Baron Cohen's character was massive. Friends said that I looked like him and so I decided to play up to it. Underneath my normal clothes I put on a yellow FUBU tracksuit, just like Ali G. A pair of shades and the famous hat went into my pockets. I was ready. When the first question came my way, I adopted an Ali G-style accent and reached for the shades and hat, then put them on. The people watching loved it!

The first year was all about allowing students to integrate into university lifestyle. There were the 59 others on my course, but also thousands studying other subjects at the university. There were the events, such as the blind date nights and the hypnosis evenings. There were the clubs and societies. I even became a member of the Afro-Caribbean Society after helping some of my new friends to choreograph a dance routine for a show. When one of their dancers dropped out on the night of the dance, I had to fill in as the only non-African-Caribbean on stage.

At first the dentistry was secondary. The modules

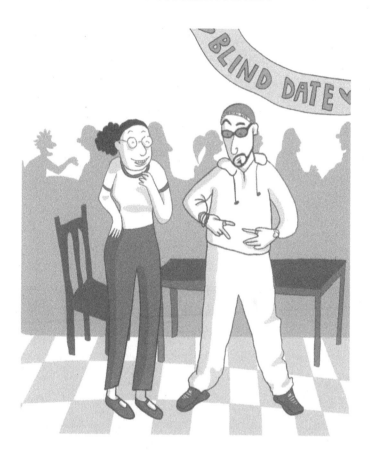

we studied were all basic introductions to topics such as oral biology, dental materials and their application, the biological structure and function of cells, and the effect of illness on people and their families. The dental school wanted us to have a holistic approach to the profession, not only teaching us the human sciences, but also aspects of sociology and psychology so we could better understand the patients we'd eventually be treating. By the fifth year, however, things became a lot more serious. The emphasis had moved from broad topics to specialised subjects to prepare us for independent practice. Communication skills were always taught and we practised this throughout the five years.

I've always liked drama and performing, so when our lecturers asked for volunteers to role-play an angry patient or a scared patient, my hand was always the first one up. During those role plays, our lecturers would reinforce the rules of communication: the importance of mirroring people, using the right tone of voice, adopting neurolinguistic programming (NLP) techniques to make the patient feel comfortable, speaking in layman's terms and avoiding overly scientific words. Communication skills help you get into dental school, but ultimately, it's an art that can be learnt.

It's said that you learn from mistakes, and some of the most memorable stories from dental school are the mistakes we all made – especially in the early days. Just like students at medical school, we learnt by practising on real live patients – who were only told about these mistakes on a need-to-know basis! A guy in the year above me called Max told me a story about the terrible mix-up that occurred when he made his first set of dentures.

There's a very set process when making dentures. First, you have to mockup a set of teeth. We use pink wax to mimic the gum, then put fake teeth into the wax before trying it in the patient's mouth to see if it looks right and proves comfortable. If not, we can melt the wax and move the teeth about until everyone is happy. Then, that mock set of teeth is taken to the laboratory so it can be turned into plastic dentures.

However, Max was in a bit of a hurry and he accidentally let the patient go home with the set of wax modelled teeth he'd produced, thinking that they were the finished item.

The next day the patient came back to reception with this pink gooey lump of teeth in his hands. 'What is it?' the receptionist asked.

'I only had a cup of tea and all my teeth fell out!' he replied.

That patient, it would turn out over my years at dental school, was actually quite lucky. It was definitely better to have been treated by Max than by student X, who shall remain nameless! Student X achieved notoriety at dental school on the day he needed to take an impression from a volunteer patient. He went to collect the impression material from the storeroom but a small mishap occurred. Student X wasn't aware that the name of the impression material he was after is very similar to the name of a dental cement. So similar that they can easily be confused. As a dental student, it was your responsibility to go to the storeroom and collect your own instruments and materials to use in clinic. So off he ran. The cement was collected by student X, who then raced back to his volunteer patient. He set about loading the material onto the tray and then moulding it around the patient's teeth. He thought he was creating an impression. That was until it came to removing the tray from the patient's mouth. Try as he might, student X couldn't get it to budge. Fear crept in. Something wasn't right.

'What did you use?'

Suddenly the tutor was at student X's side, peering into the patient's mouth. Student X told him, and the tutor's eyes widened.

'That's not the impression material!' he replied. 'That's the cement!'

If the tutor's eyes had been wide, student X's were

now wider. He watched on as the tutor put his hand inside the patient's mouth and tried to yank out the tray. Nothing. It wouldn't move. There was only one thing for it.

By now, you can imagine the patient was having second thoughts about volunteering his mouth for use by dental students. By and large, volunteer patients receive a very high level of treatment. Students have to follow everything by the book and the tutor regularly checks their work – every single stage of which has to be signed off. The volunteer patient gets the whole thing for free. They just have to pay with their time; a procedure that usually takes 15 minutes at a practice takes around two hours at dental school. But when the procedure involves the student accidentally cementing a tray to your mouth, it takes even longer. Slightly flustered, the tutor reached for his drill and set about carefully drilling the tray of cement from the patient's mouth. It was slow work, drilling the cement, then breaking it, then drilling it, then breaking it again. After three hours of drilling, the structure eventually came loose. Student X achieved legendary status after that. Thankfully, the patient walked away with everything intact.

Big up to all those volunteer patients! Without

you guys, dental students wouldn't have anybody to learn their craft and practise on – except each other.

In the early days of dental school, this is what happens. Well, after we've done a bit of practice on oranges, or something similar. We were given oranges to work on to learn how to inject a syringe, for example. Once we'd all learnt how to do that, we were split into pairs and told to stick our syringes in each other's mouths. After those weeks with the oranges, everyone was keen to get to work, but also slightly bricking it about their partner being let loose in their mouth. It soon became apparent that it was better to inject your partner first and be nice to them. That way they were more likely to be nice back with their injection. If you messed up and put your partner in pain, they'd make sure you knew about it when they got their chance for payback. For some reason, they always scheduled those syringe sessions to take place just before lunch. Our whole group would end up with super-numb mouths and spend the whole lunchtime dribbling.

After syringes, we were taught to make impressions in pairs (hands up who wants to partner up with student X!). You load up a tray and then stick it in your

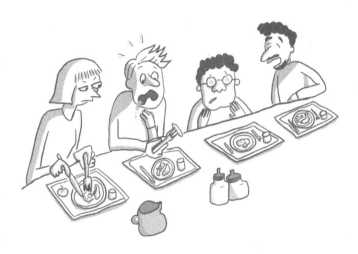

partner's mouth. When you're still learning and don't have much experience, you tend to overload the tray. That puts too much weight on, which in turn tests the gag reflexes of your partner. When Dipen loaded the tray in my mouth for the first time I thought it was heading straight down my throat and into my stomach. I wanted to throw up! Some handled it better, though. You could almost see one of the student's tonsils on their partner's impression!

As we became more experienced, we moved on to making field trips to specialist clinics to learn the more niche areas of dentistry. A colleague of mine recalls a time that he attended a clinic that specialised in jaw joint problems:

> The professor at this clinic always kept his mask on throughout the consultation. There was a small row of audience benches and an even smaller audience – just three of us: me, a younger dental student and a visiting professor from Japan. We watched as the professor had the same conversation over and over again with a stream of patients who came in with jaw problems.
>
> 'Chop up your food smaller.'
>
> 'Don't open your mouth wide.'
>
> 'Do these exercises.'
>
> 'Wear these appliances.'
>
> Done.
>
> Towards the end of the day, the most beautiful woman came in. She sat down in the chair and the professor gave her the same spiel.
>
> Only this time the patient said, 'No, I can't do that.'
>
> 'Yes, of course you can,' the professor assured her. 'It's really quite simple. Just chop up your food and take smaller mouthfuls.'

'No, I can't,' she replied. 'You can't chop up everything in your mouth to make it smaller . . . what about fellatio?'

Behind his mask, the professor's face dropped so fast he practically hit his chin on the desk. After a long silence, the visiting professor from Japan shouted, 'What fellatio, what fellatio? . . . is it a medical thing?'

Now, you might have thought that after all that effort to get into dentistry school, I let my music dream fade away so I could concentrate on my vocation. But I didn't. After moving to East London to study at Queen Mary, I carried on grinding in the South London radio scene and performing all over the city. Garage had become my number one love.

In 1999, I wrote and produced a track called 'The Vibe', and a local, more well-known MC – MC Checkers – took me under his wing. We self-released the track, made the vinyls, got a distribution deal and started to get public appearances in clubs to perform it. I was having the time of my life! All while I was a first year in dental school. Big up MC Checkers.

I had another friend who was my partner DJ. We were on the radio together and we were the sickest duo! Just like DJ Jazzy Jeff and The Fresh Prince, except we were called DJ Blackjack and MC Triple-X . . . yes, my MC name was Triple-X . . . LOL . . . Big up Blackjack. We are still best mates to this day, by the way, 22 years later!

During the third year of dental school, I started a group. We were all Iranian guys and gals with a similar look and called ourselves Goodfellaz. Big up Rembrandt, Sparkle, Lexi and my partner in rhyme, Envy! Our songs started to get played and before we knew it, we'd been offered a record deal. It was a single deal, a good offer, but my dad encouraged me to turn it down. My focus, he reasoned, should be on dentistry. I'd worked too hard on my studies to quit dental school now. The music could wait.

But . . .

I really wanted to take it.

I had to take it.

Sorry, Dad.

The label jetted us off to Ayia Napa for three weeks of performances that summer. It was an amazing experience, so exciting for a group of youngsters finding their way on a new path. Unfortunately, garage was starting to become less popular commercially and as the deal was only a single deal, an extension wasn't forthcoming. And then when garage music began to morph into grime, I decided to finally take a step back and focus on dentistry. I still kept up with my music, though. I went down a hip-hop route, doing music for fun and remixing tracks for mates. Envy and I even started a duo rap group and made a music video. It still makes me smile when I think about those times!

And so it was that in 2004, I qualified from Queen Mary and Westfield, St Barts and The London School of Medicine and Dentistry and started working in a practice in Basingstoke. It had taken a lot of sweat (mine), blood (not mine, mostly patients with gum disease) and tears (mine, the patients', my parents' and pretty much those of everyone involved in my life), but finally I was an actual proper dentist.

Young, full of energy and eager to begin my exciting new career, I couldn't wait for my first patient.

I remember the day well. As he walked in, the nerves and excitement hit me all at once. Then he opened his mouth and said it.

"Mate, I hate dentists!"

Lovely. Nice one, Milad. Your life as a dentist has begun. Looks like all the hard work has paid off.

In that moment, I wished I'd picked up a tennis ball when I was that chubby little baby in Iran. Everyone loves Roger Federer!

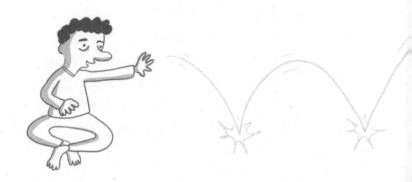

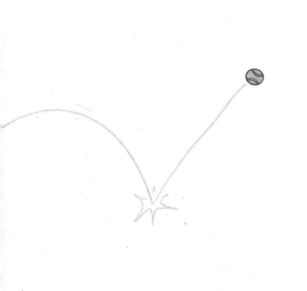

4

DENTISTRY BACKSTAGE

There's Angela on reception, Hayley on suction and Dr Milad Shadrooh on vocals. Welcome to dentistry backstage.

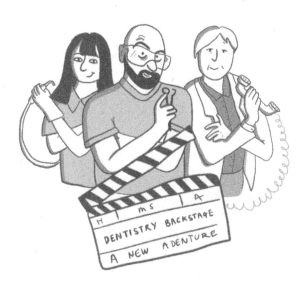

To most people, a dental clinic is somewhere they go for half an hour or so a couple of times a year. They turn up, sign in at reception, spend some time in the waiting room, then go in for their appointment. They rinse, spit and gargle, then go back down to reception and book in their next check-up. But there's so much more that goes on at a dental clinic.

At my clinic, a typical day begins at 7:45 in the morning when the first team member arrives. Usually, it will be a nurse or one of my reception team. My clinic is a friendly, long-standing practice with a homely vibe in the centre of Basingstoke. It is based in a converted Victorian terrace and we often have up to four generations of the same family on the patient list. I have been there for 16 years now and for some of my patients, I am the only dentist they have even seen! They came to me aged two sitting on their mother's lap and now they are taller than me and heading off to university. Cavity free might I add . . .

So back to the daily routine. First off, after greeting everyone in the staff room, I have to change out of my street clothes and into my scrub trousers and infamous blue tunic. I can't be doing treatments looking as if I'm fresh off the catwalk – yes, I do dress that well. At this point some dental practices like to gather their staff together for a morning huddle. It's an American thing that's caught on here; essentially a pep talk of positivity about how we're all going to CRUSH THE DAY!! Cue lots of high-fives and whooping and hollering . . . but not for us.

To actually crush the day, I need to know what's ahead. That's the beauty of dentistry. You can't just be on automatic pilot and repeat each day, because each day is different. And so I head straight up to my surgery, where Hayley's already in doing her own preparations for what's to come.

Hayley is my dental nurse, she is quiet but bubbly and very Welsh. So Welsh, in fact, that on the occasions where she's been on reception, we've had patients complimenting us on how polite our Chinese receptionist is . . . No, I'm not sure how either.

As dentists, we rely on our dental nurses utterly. Look at what happens to Maverick without Goose in *Top Gun*. Every top pilot needs a top co-pilot. In dentistry, the nurse prepares for each appointment and a good one begins to form a telepathic relationship with their dentist. The nurse knows what the dentist is going to need before they've even asked for it. I've been lucky to work with some fantastic nurses and I've experienced this first hand. I will be explaining to the patient what I'm about to do and out of the corner of my eye, I can see Hayley preparing the suction, selecting the right materials for that procedure and getting ready to rumble. Nurses can even provide support to the patients by helping to calm them down, holding their hands if they are nervous, offering soothing words in the walk from reception to the dental chair . . . trust me, a great nurse can make the practice shine.

Along with the dental nurse, one of the most important members of staff at any practice is the receptionist. You thought I was going to say dentist, didn't you? Well, of course, the dentist is super important but if the reception staff aren't any good at what they do, patients wouldn't even get to see the dentist! Receptionists play a vital role in any dental practice. When they take phone calls, they have to assess and triage every patient they speak to. They often have to give a nervous patient the confidence to book in for an appointment.

For this reason, as far as possible at our practice, we have receptionists who are also dental nurses. Having that dental knowledge, they are able to give great advice and triage effectively. The person who currently heads up our reception team is Angela, and she takes everything in her stride. Hayley, and the other nurses, work on reception too. They are all fantastic at what they do and having that nursing background really works for us. After all, a receptionist is the first person that a patient hears when they contact the practice, the first person they see when they enter and the last person they see as they leave.

Part of reception's role is to prepare the list of patients that the dentists are due to see each day. As my computer boots up, I scan the names from top to bottom. I've been at my clinic for so long that I know pretty much all the patients I see on a first-name basis. 'Oh, that's nice,' I think, as I see various names on the list. 'I wonder how they've been getting on.'

I'm not going to lie, though. There are a few – only a few! – names where you think, 'Oh gosh, they're a talker. That is NOT going to be a 15-minute appointment!'

Seeing the names and preparing myself for the procedures and patients to come helps me to visualise the day ahead and start planning. There are periods when dentists have a lot of routine care to carry out, such as check-ups. There are days when we have back-to-back treatments. Sometimes, treatments can be sandwiched between check-ups. I find it better that way. The intensity level of carrying out a treatment is very high. If a dentist does filling work or a long period of root canal work, they're having to perform intricate, delicate movements on a very small scale. It's tiring on a dentist's hands, eyes and also posture because they end up being stuck in the same position for a long period of time – sometimes several hours. If I ever have multiple lengthy treatments in a day, I know it's going to be taxing. I ask for there to be three or four 15-minute-long check-ups or review appointments either side of long treatments so I can have a break from looking at a tiny section of the mouth and work on a

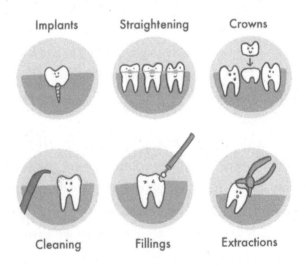

Implants   Straightening   Crowns

Cleaning   Fillings   Extractions

broader scale. Dentists need variety. I even know some dentists who arrange their appointments so they have all the trickier procedures, like root canal treatment, early on in the day. That way they aren't having to do the intricate work when they're getting a bit more tired towards the end of the day.

At our clinic, we do all sorts of procedures: check-ups, hygiene cleanings, veneers, braces and restorative work. Restorative work includes essential treatments, like using fillings to treat patients with cavities and decay, as well as more complicated procedures, such as implant work, dentures and bridges (where you replace a missing tooth by bridging the gap between the teeth with two or more anchoring crowns). We also do root canals when teeth get infected, and we carry out dental extractions when there is absolutely no alternative and the tooth is unrestorable, or the gum condition around the tooth is just too far gone. Much of the restorative work requires a good lab to fabricate the prosthetic, whether it is a denture or crown. That process can take a few days or up to two weeks. Digital dentistry, however, makes the whole process quicker. More and more practices are now using digital dentistry technology such as 3D printers and in-house milling machines to make crowns, dentures, veneers, aligners and retainers. These can then be ready for use in just a couple of hours, giving a whole new meaning to the phrase 'same-day dentistry'. The future is unfolding before our eyes, and once the cost comes down, you can expect to see this technology in all practices up and down the country.

Back to my day . . . today I don't have any root canal treatments. It doesn't look to be too taxing. If anything, it looks less taxing than usual. There are an awful lot of check-ups with . . . an awful lot of families. Slowly, the realisation dawns on me.

'Hayley, what day is it?' I ask.

'It's Monday,' she replies breezily.

'No, I mean, is it a school day today?'

'No, it's half-term this week.'

Half-term.

Oh god. Things just got a lot more chaotic.

Half-term weeks always creep up on me. I forget they're coming and then boom, there are 40 school children appointments scheduled in my diary. I like the hustle and bustle, love having families around my surgery, but I just know it's going to be carnage in the waiting room!

With the new knowledge that it's half-term week, my mental preparation takes a bit longer this morning.

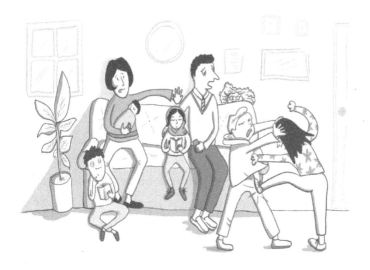

Hayley takes it all in her stride, though, and carries on preparing for all the appointments to come. She's already got the room prepped and cleaned, checked on any lab work that may have come and collected the instruments we'll need for the day ahead from central storage. Now she's getting the trays ready for each patient with all the equipment needed for the procedure they are booked in for. 'OK, so we've got this, this and this patient,' she tells me, fully focused. 'Oh, and don't forget to send off Maggie's referral and call back Robbie about his issue.'

What would I do without her?

The clock ticks to 7:59. We do one final sweep of the equipment, make sure we're loaded up and that PPE (personal protective equipment) is in place and then it's SHOWTIME.

The patients start coming in from 8am. Each slot is timed to the minute, but timetables are rarely stuck to. Running late is an occupational hazard of dentistry. Dental surgeries are about as punctual as Northern Rail. It's not pleasant but it can't be helped. We have the same problems as a GP practice or a hospital visit. However, patients don't pay for the GP or the hospital visit. They pay for their dentistry and so they expect punctuality, which isn't always possible. That's because stuff happens. What about Bertha whose dog has just died? She's my 8am appointment but she wants to tell me and Hayley exactly how it died, where it was buried and what the funeral was like. She's still tearful. You can't just shut her up, do her check-up, give her a quick clean, then move her along as soon as her time is up. No, the best dentists don't just look at teeth; they care about the human that is attached to the teeth.

The same goes for Tim, my 8:15 appointment who isn't able to come in until 8:27am. I hear him before I see him. Or, more specifically, I hear his kids before I see them. Their footsteps pound the stairs as they charge up to my surgery and then they're right in front of me in a blur of limbs. I hold out my hand for our customary high-five and they slap their palms against mine. Tim follows, looking slightly worn already. I ask his children which one wants to go first and they both stick their hands up in the air. Tim suggests the younger one goes first and the older one looks a little miffed. The younger one jumps up and asks me to let her ride the chair straight away. While I look inside her mouth, Tim tells me all about how his eldest has just passed his music exam. Tim is so proud, and when Tim is proud, he likes to talk. A lot. Time ticks on, the check-up has long since finished, but just like Bertha, I can't boot them all out of my room. I need to listen, to build rapport and trust so that my patients feel comfortable in my presence. Sometimes, however, they can feel too comfortable . . .

Later that morning a patient comes in suffering from toothache. He's been in the wars a bit and has recently had surgery on his groin. Naturally, I ask him about it as all dentists need to be aware of their patients' medical history. Everyone likes to talk about their mishaps and he tells me about his groin issues with pleasure. Satisfied that I've got everything I need from him to build up a complete medical history, I ask him to show me which tooth was hurting.

Only, he mishears me.

Before I know what's happening, he stands up straight and drops his trousers. And his pants. Nothing is left to the imagination. 'It was this one,' he tells me. I'll give him his due, though, that was an impressive groin scar.

Anyway, time runs on and before you know it, you've only got a 15-minute break at lunchtime to try and desperately shovel some limp cheese sandwiches between your molars while you compare mornings with your other staff members.

Most days, I walk with Hayley to the staff room, where I change out of my tunic and put on my civilian clothes again. Hayley's already telling Angela and Brenda about the morning's events. Brenda rolls her eyes and laughs like she's seen it all before. Which, to be fair, she probably has. Brenda is our most senior team member. In her seventies, she's been in the profession long enough to have seen a huge evolution. She comes from the era of having to mix metal fillings by hand. When she did that, the mercury would come out of the mixture and go all over her fingers. As dentistry has evolved, Brenda has had to adapt with it.

That's what makes her such a good team member. Right now, it's digital dentistry that's changing the profession. I wouldn't be surprised if I turn up one day to see Brenda all over the 3D printer like a rash! When Brenda tells a story from yesteryear, ears prick up and we sit around and listen.

My first appointment of the afternoon is an emergency patient. Emergency patients call first thing in the morning and tell the receptionist about their issue. It's then down to her to attempt to triage them on the phone, and if she can't sort the issue out, she will find space for them in our schedule. Now the patient is in my doorway and it seems he needs calming down. 'I'm a rapper and I'm shooting the music video for my new track tomorrow but my crown has fallen off!' he blurts out. Hayley passes over her pre-arranged tray and I invite the patient into the chair so I can take a look. I've had plenty of emergency patients in the past, some of them, like this one, well known. As I reach for my instruments, I'm reminded of the boxer who'd fought at both Olympic and Commonwealth level and urgently needed a gum shield. When you're an elite boxer, you can't just go and pick up a gum shield from your local sports shop. It has to be perfectly moulded. Boxers need two gum shields in case one gets

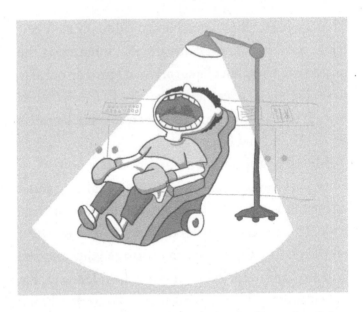

lost. Without a gum shield, you aren't allowed to fight. This boxer had a fight just a few days away but had managed to lose both his gum shields. We had to take the impressions, send them off to be made and then produce them within 24 hours. Once he had them, he had to check he was happy and able to spar in them. When someone's very career is on the line, you have to do everything in your power to squeeze them in. Plus it's pretty handy to have a boxer who owes you a favour . . .

I look inside the rapper's mouth and see that the crown hasn't fallen off, but has fully broken at the gum. It's going to require more work than the 15-minute slot he's booked in on. But it has to be fixed. There's no option but to ask the rapper to lie back in my chair and look up at the fish tank I've got playing on the screen on the ceiling. I play it to produce a calming, peaceful effect. Much of the room is geared in the same way. The chair is the first thing you see, right in front of the door. There are cabinets on either side, one set to house all the materials and instruments, the other with the computer system and drilling equipment. Windows allow plenty of natural light in. Not all dental surgeries have windows. We're lucky as ours let in a lot of natural light, which is especially important when doing cosmetic work as it increases visibility. I'll often ask patients to go and stand by the window once I'm done so I can see how their new smile looks in the real world.

I've been in this room ever since I qualified and it feels like home. I know where everything is. I enjoy my surroundings. On the rare occasions when I have to work elsewhere, everything feels awkward and weird.

The rapper sits back and watches the virtual fish swim around their virtual tank. Everyone reacts differently when they get in the chair. Some will ask you to put a DVD in so they can zone out to their favourite film – especially if it's a long appointment. Others zone out so much that they end up falling asleep. That's fine, so long as they fall asleep with their mouths open. Most of my patients, though, like to interact with me. A number of them even ask me to sing to them! 'Return of the Plaque' or 'I Like Your Molars Molars' tend to be the most requested. The rapper has no desire to hear my own rap, however. He opts to zone out and look at the fishes.

With the crown sorted, it's back to my planned afternoon of check-ups and appointments, but now we are already running late. Once again, it's mainly families. The Smiths bound up to my room, the children fizzing with energy from what I suspect to be the bottles of Fruit Shoot in their hands. I tell Mrs Smith about the danger of sugar at every appointment. Each time she smiles and nods and then gives her children a bag of Haribos as a well done. I'm going to be fighting a long-term battle with sugar and the Smiths. Still, they make me laugh. Families in general at the dental practice make me laugh. I like to get families into my surgery all together. I invite the parents to sit on the chair at the side and then ask the kids who wants to go first. Sometimes all of them put their hands up in the air; other times none of them do. There are times when one of the kids has never been to the dentist before and so they're a bit apprehensive. To encourage them, I'll invite their older sibling into the chair so they can see it isn't that scary. After that, I'll put them in the chair and let them have a ride up and down, jump around and then give them the sunglasses to put on. I might count their teeth but beyond that there's no actual dentistry. If they're really apprehensive, then we'll let them sit on the chair in their parent's lap. Everything depends on the personality of the child.

Personality is one thing that the Smiths aren't short of. 'Have you been brushing twice a day?' I ask the older one of the siblings. 'Yes, they have,' Mrs Smith replies so quickly I wonder how she even heard the end of my sentence.

'No, we don't,' says the younger Smith. 'I hate brushing!'

That's what I love about working with kids. As Mrs Smith looks daggers at her younger child, I can't help but smile. Kids are so honest. When I treat adults they might not like going to the dentist but they just get in the chair and put up with it. With children, if they don't want to do something, there's no way you can force them to do it. I've seen all kinds of strops and

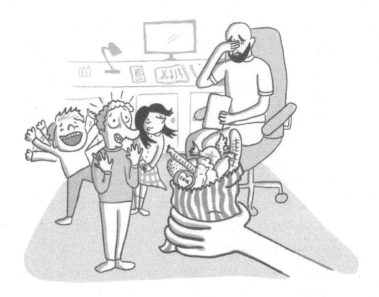

stubbornness in my surgery. That's fine. A dentist shouldn't push a young patient to do something they don't want to in case it turns into a traumatic experience for them. Maybe they're having the strop because it's the first time they've been in this strange-looking room with this bloke in a blue tunic with his upside-down head. Maybe they're just having a bad day. In those instances, I just let them get used to being in the room and have a chat to their parent or guardian to give general dental advice, then give them a sticker. If they truly are fearful, each appointment is about building their confidence so that they learn the ropes and eventually feel comfortable enough for me to look in their mouth.

With the Smiths there was never any apprehension. I start with the older one, while the younger one charges around the room like he's racing in the Grand Prix. I let him crack on. Mrs Smith can deal with that. The older one opens his mouth and I look inside. Not bad, considering the lack of brushing. This will be a routine check-up. As I look around the mouth, I'm reminded of a story from a former colleague.

He worked as a dental hygienist for 23 years and early on in his career he was temping at an office. A patient came in for a routine check-up, which required some X-rays to be taken. For these specific X-rays, the patient has to bite a cardboard tab to keep them in place. Only this patient didn't find it so easy to bite. You see, she had a terrible gag reflex. The solution, the dentist thought, was simple. He picked up his trusty topical anaesthetic and sprayed it in the back of the patient's mouth. He'd done it hundreds of times before and never had any problems.

AAAARRRRRGGGGGHHHHHHHHH!!!

The patient's eyes were popping out of her head, her body writhing around in the chair.

Talk about dramatic.

A second round of spray should do it.

Again, a dramatic reaction. This time, an involuntary dry mist emerged from the patient's mouth. 'That's weird,' the dentist thought. Still, he managed to get the X-ray so the topical obviously worked.

Once the patient's appointment was over and the usual future check-ups arranged, the dentist decided to take a second look at the spray.

Oh god.

No wonder the patient had reacted in that way.

That wasn't topical anaesthetic spray. It was endo ice, usually used to check the nerve fibres of the teeth. Who wouldn't have reacted that way if they'd had minus 30 degrees of cold sprayed all around their mouth?

But at least it got the job done!

The older Smith gets sent off the chair and then I examine the younger one's mouth while Hayley takes notes. With both siblings signed off, the Smiths are good to go. Mrs Smith will come back another time for herself. She couldn't possibly leave her two little ones to their own devices while she was in the chair. I give her children stickers and they look thrilled, though not quite as thrilled as if they'd got lollipops. Many of my patients still expect to get a lollipop at the end of their appointment as in the old days, even though I've told them how damaging sugar is. There aren't many dentists now who'll give lollipops – in fact, I don't know any – but there are certain professions that do give you them. Barbers are notorious for it; and there's still the odd GP who has a tray load of them. GPs used to be synonymous with lollipops back in the day. I don't know if there was some kind of backdoor agreement between GPs and dentists to keep us dental professionals in business . . . The children stick their stickers proudly on their chests and Mrs Smith smiles and hands them both a bag of sweeties for their troubles. Cue eye rolls from me and Hayley and cheers from the two little ones.

The rest of the afternoon seems to be check-up after check-up, family after family. Half-term weeks are among the busiest, and keeping busy is integral to having a sustainable business: that's the main thing that differentiates dentistry from other forms of healthcare – except optometry. It has to be treated as a business. You can't operate at a loss year after year because otherwise you wouldn't be able to run a dental clinic. Doctors working in a hospital setting have one main concern – caring for their patients. The health of our patients is also essential for us. We must to do a good job to keep them healthy and happy, but we also need to ensure we do so without losing money for the practice. Therefore, we need to consider both profit and ethics at all times. Put too much resource into your patients without ensuring you make a profit and you'll go out of business. Focus too much on profit and your quality of care will inevitably suffer and your patients will leave you. The ideal balance is to work prethically. That's right. It's a new word I have heard from a dental business guru. Profitable ethics = prethics. This should be the goal for all dental clinics.

Just like any other business, a dental practice also needs to market itself – to drum up awareness and attract patients. A dentist friend of mine, Doctor Z, used to advertise his services through Google ads. It was still a new format at that time, so it was a test-and-learn approach. He wrote and designed his own advert, including a bit of information about the practice, a bit about himself, and spelled out in big letters his main interest of working as an IMPLANTOLOGIST.

It worked. There was a notable increase in the number of people booking appointments. Business was thriving. He told me about one encounter he had with a new patient:

'A new patient came in for the first time. A nice-looking, 40-year-old lady. The receptionist greeted her and then the nurse put her in the chair. I was writing my notes from the previous appointment, so I smiled at her and asked her to make herself comfortable, reassuring her that I'd be with her in just a minute. When I finished typing up the last word and turned back to face the patient, my eyes nearly popped out of their sockets. She'd pulled her top up and had her boobs out, and was asking, "So what can you do with these?"

'I didn't know what to do, I was so shocked, and for some reason, I put my hands up in the air as if it was a stick-up! Meanwhile, the patient was touching her boobs and jiggling them about. "I really need these sorted," she continued.

'Only then did it click what had happened . . . I cried out at her, "No, no, no, I do teeth. Dental implants. DENTAL implants!" After an awkward jiggle, the lady left the practice and I made a slight tweak to that advert.'

Marketing your business can occasionally give you more than you bargained for, just like it did with

Doctor Z. By and large, I've stayed away from it. The benefit of being around in the community for donkey's years is that word-of-mouth referrals are strong. We get so many people coming to us because their aunt's friend's son had a good experience during his check-up. The only time, I have ventured into the world of advertising is when we have started to provide a new cosmetic service such as facial aesthetics or teeth straightening, and even then I've limited myself to internet marketing.

As the owner of my practice, it isn't just marketing the business that takes me beyond what's expected of a dentist. It's also on me to make sure the books are balanced and my patients are receiving the best care possible. I have to pay the bills, my staff, PAYE, loans, national insurance and all sorts of other costs. In addition to that, I have to do stock checks, order materials and pay registrations and licences. I have been able to start delegating some of these tasks but still, a dental business has some unique measures that need to be in place. For example, we can't just go around the back and chuck the rubbish in a bin. We have to have special sanitary bins, for which we need to hire a special waste management company, who remove all waste safely from the premises. Bodily fluids, blood and removed teeth are all dealt with by them. I'm pretty sure it all ends up in the same rubbish dumps eventually but clinical waste must be incinerated.

Then, take the simple task of cleaning the floor. Now, I get that a practice needs to be clean. I can't put patients at risk of contracting an infection from dirty rooms. But the rules are draconian! Even for something as simple as cleaning a floor, we have to use a special cleaning product that meets certain requirements and we must have all the necessary Medical and Healthcare products Regulatory Agency (MHRA) safety documentation. It must be colour coded, kept in a specific place and registered. Cleaners have to undergo training to make sure they know how to use it properly and there are checklists to ensure that they have done so. And that's just cleaning the floor . . .

You know all those horrible-looking instruments on the stainless-steel tray? Well, all equipment needs to be cleaned after each use. We can't just put it in a washing-up bowl and give it a quick scrub. In our dental practice, we have a special decontamination room. I don't mean we need to be decontaminated . . . it's not like a sci-fi movie where we walk into a chamber and get air blasted with disinfectant. It is for all of our dental instruments.

So when my 3:30pm appointment exclaims, 'How much for a crown?! £650!' I have to count to five and remember that they aren't necessarily aware of the millions of things a dental practice needs to pay for just to stay open, let alone function! The £650 has to cover a lot more than just a bit of porcelain.

By the time my last appointment comes in, I have to give myself a mini pep talk. One more to go. It's been a long, intense day. Fortunately, Angela has sorted me out with a routine check-up – which is just as well because, thanks to all the delays, it starts five minutes before closing time. I can probably count on one hand the number of times we have finished at 5pm over the years. More smiles, more 'bye for nows', and the day's patients have all been seen. I nod at Hayley and Hayley nods at me, congratulating each other on another day's work well done. Now that the last patient has left, there's just one thing left to do: the close-down process.

Surfaces are wiped, clutter is cleared, instruments removed, autoclaves fired up, money counted, stock checked and notes completed. My main focus is on the notes, while Hayley cleans the dental area – the sides, worktops and chair – then removes and replaces the protective barriers, drains the water lines from the drill and empties the clinical waste bin. Now that I'm writing this, the jobs list does seem a bit unfair! After Hayley has done all of that she'll start preparing for the next day, making sure that we have certain instruments and materials ready. Meanwhile, Brenda is helped by another nurse, Puja, to perform all the routine checks required to shut down the decontamination room.

We all walk out of the clinic as a team. Brenda hits the lights and locks the door, and we pile out into the street.

'What a day! Wasn't it busy!'

'What's everyone doing this evening?'

'I've got a nice steak in the fridge for tonight.'

'Ooh that sounds lovely.'

'I think I'll have a glass of wine.'

'You do that, you've earned it.'

Once we're out of there, it's down to the cleaner to work their magic and prepare the practice for another day of appointments and stories from all sorts of interesting patients. Our cleaner is an important member of the team – even if we never see her! She works in all the communal areas, making sure they're spick and span for the next day's patients. Every morning when I walk in the place looks immaculate.

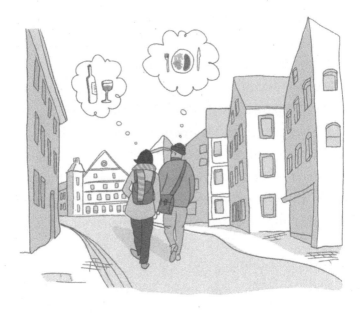

Having a place to be proud of and a team to be proud of makes everything so much easier.

It's the staff in particular that make our dental practice what it is: from the receptionists, to the nurses, to the dentists. We can't do everything by ourselves. You know why? Because *teamwork makes the dream work!*

Of course, it's not always plain sailing. We always aim to do our best for our patients, but sometimes mistakes do happen. We are all human and we cannot be 100% perfect 100% of the time. In my experience, most issues can be rectified, and the vast majority of patients are understanding and just want things fixed.

However, this is not always the case. In recent years, many have become increasingly litigious. Some like to sue for anything. Toothache after seeing the dentist? Sue. Teeth are still yellow? Sue. Misdiagnosed? Sue. This can start to explain why these days most dentists pay an average of £8000 for dental insurance. I even have friends who have to pay as much as £18,000 in insurance, just for the privilege of having someone come and sit in their dental chair. Cosmetic dentistry commands some of the highest insurance premiums. If a patient does make a complaint, it can be deeply upsetting. Even if it is totally outrageous and you know there is no merit in the complaint, it is still something that plays on your mind and can cause immense stress. You may have done everything by the book, but one element didn't go well and now you are being accused of being terrible at your job and having a negative impact on your patient's life. This is a lot of pressure to deal with. It only takes one case to ruin all the years of good work you have done. This is a key factor contributing to the alarming suicide rate among dentists, one of the highest of any profession.

The good news is that many of the other changes

we've seen recently in dentistry have been overwhelmingly positive. Dentists are excited to see where digital dentistry is taking us, and the enhanced materials being created through computer-aided design and other innovations, which are helping to improve people's smiles. The main change I've found has been in our patients. Their level of understanding seems to improve every year. When I first started as a dentist, it would be the patient asking me what I thought was best. Now, it's more common that a patient tells me what they want. That comes from aesthetic awareness, which in turn comes from the exposure of millions of smiles on social media, film and TV – in particular reality shows. Patients' role models have white straight teeth, so that's what they want too. They understand that there's a financial transaction involved. If they're investing money, they want their smile to be perfect. They stare and stare at their teeth in the mirror and even notice the tiniest imperfection. Understanding has improved, and consequently expectation has heightened. Patients are much more engaged with the dental process, and that can only be a positive thing.

Over the years, I've had all kinds of people in my practice. The dental chair doesn't discriminate. My patients have brought with them all kinds of stories. Some have made me smile, others have honestly made me cry, while plenty have made my jaw drop.

Isn't that the beauty of dentistry?

5

THE BIRTH OF THE
SINGING DENTIST

From the start, while working at my dental practice, I have had to do my best to squeeze the musical side of my life into whatever precious free time I have been able to find. Back in 2004, when I qualified as a dentist, my ex-partner Envy had become a big boy promoter. He gave me a shot at DJing at his events, and it was the buzz I was looking for. An outlet for the musical energy I couldn't get rid of. As a result, I got into DJing properly, buying the equipment and spending hours refining and making tunes to play.

I even DJed at my wedding, something my wife was thrilled about! I also managed to get a weekly residency in a club close to home, so on Saturday night, I was smashing it from 10pm to 3am, spinning records for fun. Then my daughter was born. My wife didn't mind me taking up *her* time with my DJing, but we both agreed I couldn't do the same to our little girl. Every Sunday would be a write-off as I attempted to recover from the night before.

The solution was to slowly phase out the DJing. But I still had this urge, this musical talent and vibe and energy – what could I do? I continued to drop freestyle raps and send them round to my mates, but was it enough? That's when The Singing Dentist was born.

After that first DIY video of me channelling Drake's song went viral, it got me thinking.

If the general public liked and shared my first song, then surely I had to ride that wave of popularity. What could I do next? How could I build momentum? The obvious decision was to parody the song of the moment which, at the time, was 'Happy' by Pharrell Williams.

Happy . . . happy . . . happy . . . what could I do? How could I make it about dentistry?

Gappy? Hold on. That could work. If you don't brush your teeth, then you're going to end up gappy. If you don't floss your teeth, you're going to end up gappy.

Hahaha. There it was. This time I wanted to do things differently, though. There had been some really specific dental terminology in the first freestyle. The general public doesn't know what an *endo* is. I wanted to strip all that specific terminology out of the parody and make it accessible to the average person on the street. I would use layman's terms for everything and give a bit of light-hearted advice around oral hygiene.

This might seem crazy what I'm 'bout to say
But as a dentist I see this every day
You know, patients aren't worried if their
gums bleed
Don't you know, that could be a sign of gum
disease?
And you know, you might be gappy
If you don't brush your teeth for two minutes
twice a day
You might be gappy
If you don't floss your teeth to clean all
that plaque away
You might be gappy
If you're smoking 20 a day, then try to cut
down please
You might be gappy
If you lose all your teeth because of gum disease

Now you can prevent gingivitis
Yeah!
Just book an appointment with a hygienist
Yeah!
They will scale your teeth and get right in between
Yeah!
And they will help you improve your oral hygiene
And if you don't, well
You might be gappy
If you don't brush your teeth for two minutes
    twice a day
You might be gappy
If you don't floss your teeth to clean all that plaque
    away
You might be gappy
If you're smoking 20 a day then, try to cut
    down please
You might be gappy
If you lose all your teeth because of gum disease
And we don't wanna see you gappy, gappy,
    gappy!

This time I wasn't going to rely on Dr Payman to share my work with the wider world. The video was going to be uploaded on my terms. But first I'd need a

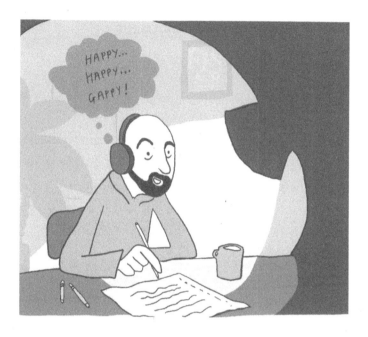

name. I couldn't share my work as Dr Milad. No, I needed a proper stage name.

What could I call myself?

Well, I reasoned, I'm a dentist, and I rap. Put two and two together and you get The Rapping Dentist. Jokes! It made so much sense. Rap was my background and I was doing parodies of rap songs.

I designed a logo. My eyebrows had attracted loads of positive comments in the 'Hotline Bling' parody so I made them the centre point, drawing a cartoon style version of my face with prominent brows. 'Rapping' went above the drawing and 'Dentist' below.

Voila.

I was good to go. First, though, I wanted to run it by someone. Someone close to me.

'Dad, I put a video out and people seem to like it. I'm going to upload another one. What do you think of this logo I'm going to use?'

He studied the logo, then studied it a bit closer, frowning a little. 'What is this Raping Dentist?'

What?!

'Dad! It's two ps. Rapping. Rapping.'

'No, no, no. Other people will think the same. Call yourself Singing Dentist instead.'

For the record, I'm not sure many others would have made the same mistake but you don't say no to your dad, do you? He told me about this iconic character from way back called The Singing Detective. If the name worked for him, and my dad still remembered him all these years later, he thought it might just work for me. No matter how many times I tried to tell Dad that I couldn't sing, he refused to hear any other option.

OK. I started to come around to his way of thinking. Maybe it wasn't the worst idea. The fact that I couldn't sing and was always out of tune might actually be pretty funny. I got the logo back up on my screen and changed 'Rapping' to 'Singing'.

Then I clicked upload. The 'Gappy' video was out there on The Singing Dentist's official YouTube channel. Straight away I shared it on all my social channels and texted it to my mates, and almost immediately the view count shot upwards. 300,000. 400,000. 500,000 views. Crazy!

So much love. So many amazing comments. 'You've made toothbrushing fun.' 'My kids brush their teeth now because of you.' 'I used to hate dentists.' 'You've reminded me that seeing the dentist isn't bad.'

This couldn't be a one-off or a two-off. This had to become a thing.

MJ was the next artist to receive the Singing Dentist treatment. 'Oh you wanna be starting something' became 'Oh you wanna do some teeth whitening'. Again, loads of love, so when 'Cheerleader' by OMI came out, I parodied the lyrics to 'Oh I think that I found myself a sweet eater'.

Little did I know that my dental nurse had alerted the local paper, the *Basingstoke Gazette*, to my videos. She'd told them about all the amazing comments and how much people seemed to like my parodies. The same afternoon they came to the practice with the intention of running a feature article. They interviewed me, took a few pictures, and the next day it went out in the paper.

That article was picked up by a big Southampton-based news organisation that shared it with other papers. Twenty-four hours after the first article, the *Metro* published a piece. It being a free newspaper, my mates suddenly sat up and took notice. The cheapskates!

The *Metro* article was massive for me, though. So many influential people read that paper – and suddenly I was being asked to do all sorts of interviews. First to the phone was BBC News, then ITV London asked me to come into their studios to do their Friday story. I jumped on the very first train I could, and later that evening I watched myself back on the telly. Mum, I made it!

And that was only the start. Two weeks later, Lorraine was talking about my videos with Dr Hilary. Their amazing medical story of the week was The Singing Dentist. Lorraine told Dr Hilary that he could be The Singing Doctor. Now, now, there can be only one!

The next week Dr Hilary couldn't make it to the

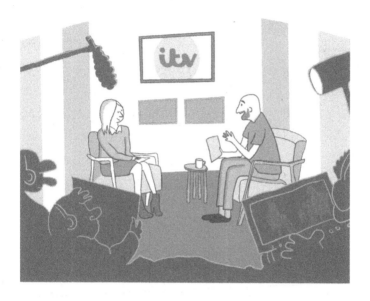

studio. Maybe he actually was training to become the Singing Doctor? Whatever it was, they needed a replacement.

An unknown number popped up on my phone. Wondering whether I was about to be sold PPI or if I'd been in a recent accident that wasn't my fault, I clicked accept. But it wasn't an automated robot on the other end. It was ITV. They wanted me to come in as Dr Hilary's replacement and do a piece on dentistry. *Live*.

I'd never done live TV before. I'd barely even done TV before. And yet here I was, due to be broadcast to millions of people. The segment ended up being six minutes long. There was a phone-in and then I was invited to bust some popular myths. I didn't make any bloopers or swear on air or anything. And I must have done OK, because a few days later *Good Morning Britain* called. 'There's a story about child tooth decay. Would you like to come into the studio and talk about it?'

The TV appearances kept on coming. I established myself as ITV's go-to dentist. Whenever there was a story about teeth, I'd get a phone call. All the while, I was creating more and more parodies. 'Return of the Plaque' came to me while I was DJing and I dropped 'Return of the Mack' by Mark Morrison. I wrote the lyrics in my head and then recorded it the next morning. Now that I was becoming better known, big content pages such as LADBible were sharing my videos and getting me some serious viewing figures: 15,000,000 views for 'Return of the Plaque' and 8,000,000 for 'I Like Your Molars Molars'.

The biggest hit, though, was my Ed Sheeran parody. When 'Shape of You' came out, I'd actually cut down on my parody output to avoid becoming a bit stale. I didn't want my videos to start being boring. After all, how many times can you tell people to brush their teeth and not eat sweets? But Ed's comeback was so big, that I felt I just had to do something. On social media, when there's a wave you jump on that wave and ride it as hard as you can. You have to try to make yourself topical. Shape of you. Shape of you. Shave your tooth? No, that doesn't sound good.

As I was wracking my brains, my wife, piped up. 'Why don't you just say save your tooth.'

Hold on. I like that.

I wrote 'Save Your Tooth' really quickly and uploaded it to my channel the same day. That's when everything really went mental. We're not just talking going-on-TV mental. We're talking conversations-backstage-with-Ed-Sheeran mental.

It seemed that every big media company shared my video. It was viewed more than 38,000,000 times. My follower count shot up from 200,000 to 500,000. News channels from all over the world were calling. Australian TV invited me on. Ellen's producers called from America and asked me to make a special parody for Ellen DeGeneres.

Somehow, Ed heard it. He was being interviewed on BBC Radio One and they asked him if he'd heard The Singing Dentist's version of his song. 'Yeah,' he replied, 'I have. It's great.'

Rahhhh.

Ed Sheeran was due to perform at a concert in aid of the Teenage Cancer Trust later that week. The organiser contacted me and invited me along. On the night of the concert, I found myself backstage at the Royal Albert Hall. My task was to perform some parodies for the Teenage Cancer Trust's guests. They seemed to enjoy my act, and one or two even told me they were more excited to meet me than Ed Sheeran! Most, though, were waiting for Ed's set. He was the highlight of the night, the last on the bill. And then there he was, walking right in front of us as he headed for the stage. He said hello to the guests, smiled at a

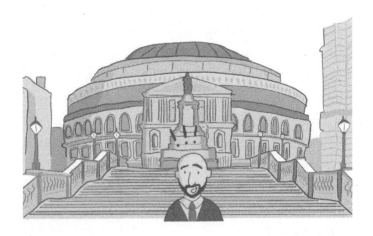

few people, then we made eye contact. He carried on walking, then did a double take. 'Hold on, you're The Singing Dentist.'

Rahhhh.

I was as weak at the knees as a little school kid. Proper fan-boy moment. 'How are you, mate?' Ed continued. 'Let's have a photo.' He put his arm around me and I tried to control my eyebrows from leaping off my face as we both smiled for the cameras. 'Mate, I'll catch up with you in a bit,' he said. 'I've just got to go on stage.'

As I stood in the Royal Albert Hall, fresh from interacting backstage with musical royalty and blown away by Ed's talent, I couldn't help but think all those years back to my school talent show, when I made my decision that performing was what I wanted to do for the rest of my life. I thought back, too, to the record deal that I was offered and my dad's determination for me to see out dental school instead. He was sure that the music could wait. He knew that I'd end up on the right path, doing what I love.

As the memories flooded back, I couldn't help but smile. Dad, you were right after all.

6

KEEPING IT SOCIAL

When I started as The Singing Dentist, social media wasn't really used in dentistry. Most dentists were more likely to down pints of sugar than share the results of their latest root canal treatment while dancing around on the internet. And with good reason. Back then, social media was still growing. YouTube was really the only place to upload videos. Facebook was all about posting on each other's walls. Instagram let you share pictures and not much else. And TikTok was the sound that a clock makes.

As those platforms developed and became more sophisticated, however, they offered more opportunity. I began to play around, doing live streams on Facebook with my followers, jumping on Snapchat, experimenting with videos on Instagram when that became a thing. And people started watching. Despite the bad rep it often gets, I realised that there really *is* an audience out there interested in dentistry.

There has always been a relationship between dentist and patient. As a patient, you go to the dentist, the dentist tells you what you need and you're probably going to accept what they tell you. The dentist knows a lot more than you and so you trust their professional opinion. It's like when I go to a mechanic to get my car fixed. I don't know how cars work and I assume that the mechanic does. The mechanic then looks at my car, gives an honest appraisal and tells me how much it's going to cost. Perhaps I'll get a second opinion from another mechanic, but I'm going to end up paying one of them to fix my car.

What's really had an impact on dentistry over the last few years, however, is the growth of social media. Patients have consumed content that educates and informs them about their mouth, their teeth and possible treatments.

That's thanks to the ever-increasing number of dentists who are establishing themselves on social media. Perhaps, in some ways, my success as The Singing Dentist has opened the door for others. There are now all sorts of The [insert word] Dentist. We've got The Cooking Dentist, The Food Dentist, The PT

Dentist, The Dancing Dentist, The Dentist Who Cares, The Holistic Dentist, The Blah Blah Blah Dentist. There are millions of them popping up and I love it! It's great to see so many dentists sharing their human side, which is ultimately what social media was created for.

Dentists share their life experience with dedicated audiences who have actively chosen to follow them and hear what they have to say. In doing so, these dentists are changing perceptions. They're helping patients to see that we aren't all stuffy and old and only here to hurt you, take all your money and then drive

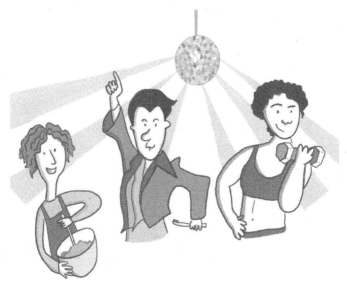

off in our Porsches. More and more patients are seeing dentists as young, dynamic, forward-thinking and entrepreneurial. They understand we care for the patient and want to practise good dentistry.

The free information that dentists have been sharing has increased patient awareness to a level beyond anything seen before. So has the growing number of patients using their own social media accounts to share experiences and photos of the successful treatments they've had. It's got to the stage where some patients come in and tell me what they want, rather than the traditional method of me having a look and telling them what they need.

'Morning, Milad, I want Invisalign followed by composite bonding please, mate,' they'll say.

Oh my god.

How do they even know this?

They know because they've researched it, they've seen the pictures from patients and dentists and they understand the results this procedure can produce. Some will even proactively contact dentists whose treatment they've seen online and ask if they can be registered for the same procedure.

In that regard, social media has armed dental practices with a powerful marketing tool. Not only through the content they post, but also through the paid advertising opportunities. With social media, dentists can target the right kind of patient with the right kind of information. Through these digital tools, dentists can then consult patients so that by the time they come in, the patient is super informed, super motivated and super excited. You then do fantastic dentistry for them and everyone is a winner. It's allowed dentists to build humongous enterprises. And it isn't just dentists and their practices that are benefiting.

Remote monitoring companies have recognised the huge potential of digital media. They now offer patients virtual consultations in which the patient uploads a set of images of their teeth and the company then teaches them how to make them perfect – all through the power of the internet.

Covid really helped speed that one along.

Then there are the direct-to-patient companies. I am not a huge fan of these as they often bypass the dentist and they've been able to grow because there are some treatments for which, strictly speaking, you don't necessarily need a dentist. Straightening teeth, for example, can be done at home. For this, a patient needs to go to one of the company's centres to have their teeth scanned by someone who isn't a dentist. The company will then assess the scans, plan all the movements and send the patient a tooth alignment pack that can be inserted at home. Throughout the whole process, a patient doesn't need to see a dentist once.

But let's think about this another way. Back to that mechanic and my car, which is knackered again . . .

This time round, I want to save a few bob. I know my car is in a bad way, but I think my best bet is to cut out the hefty chunk of money used on the specialist. I take my car to a different mechanic who has a quick look to confirm the problem. Instead of fixing it there and then, they send me a new battery in the post, along with the cam belt and the water pump, and some instructions to follow so that I can change everything at home. I do the work myself, and hope the car doesn't explode. At least I save a few quid . . .

But I don't. Chances are, the car *will* explode. It may not happen the first time I replace the cam belt – it might be on the tenth attempt – but if I do mess up, it's going to cost a lot more than I've saved on those hours of mechanic time. I'll probably need a

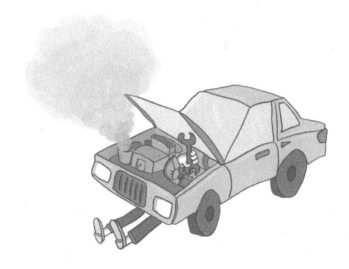

whole new engine rather than a couple of replacement parts.

Patients have information coming at them from all sides; from the new companies popping up, from dentists and patients on social media posting about their treatments, and also from reality TV stars and influencers who aren't shy about showing their shiny white teeth. When followers and viewers see these pearly whites, they often want them too.

But – and there's a big BUT here – people can't always have the treatments they want. It pains me to say it because I always want happy patients. The reality, though, is that some people's teeth just aren't suitable for certain treatments. People see influencer after influencer with perfect white teeth and think, 'if I had teeth like that, I could probably go on *Love Island*.' So they come to the dentist, only to be told, 'Sorry, that treatment isn't suitable for you' or 'That's going to cost way more money than you probably expected or budgeted for.'

But that isn't the end of the road for the patient. Social media has made the world smaller. Now patients are aware that they can get certain treatments abroad and even better, they're aware that may cost a lot less. Consequently more and more people are travelling overseas for treatment in pursuit of the perfect smile. So, they buy a return flight, head off abroad and come back with 20 brand-new, tile-white porcelain teeth that don't necessarily suit them and that their regular dentist warned against. Why did their regular dentist warn against the treatment? Well, this person is in their early twenties and the dentist has drilled all their teeth down to stumps.

Not cool.

The treatment may last for a few years, but what then? Inevitably the work is going to have to be replaced. Does the patient fly back to the same clinic?

Will the clinic even exist still? Will they have to go to a different country? And what are they actually going to do the second time round, considering their teeth have already been hacked up? We can sometimes repair the damage with new crowns, but there is always a risk that the teeth will have been irrevocably damaged.

Major celebrities are doing it. Influencers are pushing it. However, no one is thinking about what they're going to do when they're in their forties, fifties and sixties? Their teeth have already been drilled to stumps, so there's nothing left. A mouthful of extractions and dental implants is looming and it will be down to their regular dentist to pick up the pieces.

Although the growing influence of social media in dentistry has been positive in many ways, it has inevitably had its downsides too. On balance, though, the whole online world has improved dentistry and I think we're only at the beginning of the journey. Patients are now far more empowered, way more knowledgeable and way less tolerant of dentists who don't meet their expectations.

Down the line, I'm sure more patients will use social media to find dentists, develop their understanding and educate themselves. Practices will continue to expand through social media. More online tools will be created to allow for virtual consultations and the like.

Ultimately, we're all going to end up in the metaverse, mate.

7

THE BEAUTY OF TEETH

Dentistry as a profession has a surprisingly good adherence rate. Of the original 60 students in my year at dental school, 55 qualified. Of the remaining five, two had to repeat a year, while the other three took their last chance to escape dentistry by transferring to another Bachelor of Science course. When you qualify as a dentist, you almost always get a job as a dentist. Every single graduate in my year became a dentist: 55 out of 55. After a few years, some – like me – began buying practices.

My fellow graduates are still doing all sorts of diverse things in the dentistry world. Some have gone into product development and several have property portfolios. One imports equipment from abroad. Many run their own practices. But many, many more are still working full-time as dentists. Like me, they have the money and experience to lead a comfortable life but they still work incredibly hard because they love what they do. They love teeth. And who can blame them?

Teeth are fascinating. I'm not just saying that because I'm a dentist. Honestly, they are! Their role within the body is vital. The same goes for the mouth. Not convinced? Try eating a burger without using your mouth. Pretty hard, right?

Some of the world's most famous teeth belonged to Freddie Mercury, the iconic lead singer of Queen. He was blessed with four extra incisors, which created an overbite, meaning his teeth stuck out more than average. Yet he never fixed them. Despite being minted, Freddie opted to keep his teeth the way they were because he believed they gave him greater vocal range. He feared that if he changed his teeth's positioning, it would have an impact on his voice. And when you've got one of the best voices in pop history, that's quite some fear!

There's method to Mercury's beliefs. Teeth do affect the way you sing, as well as the way you talk. Lisping, for example, is predominantly to do with the position of your jaw and your teeth and how your tongue hits the inside of the teeth to make

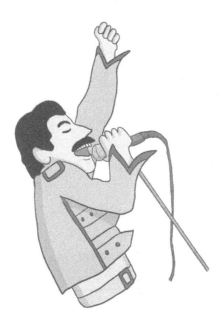

certain sounds. You make the 'T' sound by hitting your top teeth with your tongue. 'F' is pronounced by pressing your lips into your top teeth and releasing air through them. 'Ch' happens when your tongue presses against the upper side of your teeth. You get the picture. Or, if you have no teeth, you get the pic-err . . . sorry.

When children lose teeth prematurely through trauma or lack of care, their speech development is hindered. Their tongue can't always hit the right teeth to make the right noises. That can affect their confidence. They may shy away from social situations, avoid speaking in class or limit their interactions.

Speech isn't the only important function of teeth. Let's stay on the confidence angle for a minute – and I'm going to get a bit philosophical.

What's the meaning of life?

42? (In-joke for fans of *The Hitchhiker's Guide to the Galaxy* . . .)

Maybe, but to many people the meaning of life is to ensure life continues. As a species, we've been procreating ever since Adam treated Eve to a slap-up meal in the Garden of Eden. What do you think attracted Eve to Adam? OK, she didn't exactly have much choice in the matter. But if there were some other suitors in that garden, why do you think she'd have chosen Adam?

His skin?

His hair?

His nose?

The little leaf covering his dignity?

His smile?

When a person is attracted to a mate, their smile and their teeth are among the first things that they notice. Much more so than their clothes and hair, which people spend so much time and money on.

Many of the people who appeared on the Jeremy Kyle show may disprove this theory, but teeth are an essential part of the peacock ritual that comes with choosing a mate.

If you smile, you're probably going to show your teeth. If you don't have teeth, you may not have the confidence to smile. A smile can open up all sorts of lines of communication, saying a lot without saying anything at all. Think about a baby. Their smile is one of their most important means of communication. When you smile at a baby and they smile back, that's a powerful and life-enhancing connection.

What makes me smile? Sitting down at the table with a full plate of food in front of me. I love to eat. Who doesn't? Eating is, and should be, an enjoyable experience. You don't just eat for sustenance. If the only reason people ate was to stay alive then they'd just drink all their electrolytes and proteins and fats and that'd be enough to survive. If flavour and texture were not important, the process of eating would be completely different.

Imagine a succulent fillet of beef (sorry vegetarians) – a full set of teeth truly adds to the experience of eating it. I've got plenty of patients who are all gums and no teeth, and they can still chow down one, but the sensation isn't as good as it is for someone with plenty of well brushed and well flossed teeth. What about those who suffer from sensitive teeth? Eating ice cream gives them more than just brain freeze! The tooth sensitivity it can cause may force them to avoid the ice cream entirely and miss out on an amazing dessert, which is a real shame.

Why wouldn't you take proper care of your mouth? If I had a pound for every time I had to tell a patient to floss, I'd be a very, very rich dentist. Many people see it as a chore. But I see it in a different way. If you haven't already guessed, your mouth is very important. Now picture this: say you had to have a tooth removed, as a result of trauma, neglect or disease. The best replacement for a lost tooth is a dental implant, which is essentially a titanium screw inserted into the jawbone where the missing tooth used to be. This acts as the root of the tooth. We then place a crown on top of the implant, which acts as the visible part of the tooth.

That implant and crown costs, on average, £2500. £2500!

So, let me get my calculator out. Every person is blessed with 28 teeth, excluding the wisdom teeth. In some cases, other teeth may also be congenitally missing, but the majority of people will have 28, seven in each quadrant of the mouth. That's 28 lots of £2500. Twenty-eight multiplied by 2500 equals £70,000!

You are born with a mouth worth £70,000! Imagine going to your next check-up and your dentist giving you a hefty bag of cash. 'Listen, there's £70,000 in that bag – all you've got to do is look after it.'

Sounds all right, doesn't it? You're probably going to look after that money. But suppose the dentist doesn't give it to you as a bag of money. Suppose they

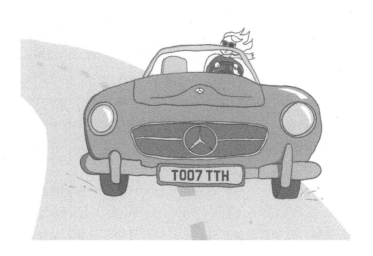

give you a piece of jewellery or a brand-new Mercedes instead. You're still probably going to look after it. You'll take your jewellery off and store it in a safe place when you're doing the washing up. You'll regularly check the oil and water in your Mercedes and take it to the car wash.

But teeth?

Nah, I'll floss tomorrow instead. I've already brushed them once today. Hold on, is that a bag of Haribo?

You wouldn't put £70,000 in a bin. Yet I end up having to remove and throw away so many teeth.

It's such a waste. Every single tooth is alive until it's removed. It has blood vessels, nerves going in and out, three different surfaces, including enamel, the hardest structure in your body, and ligament wrapped around it to anchor it to the bone and act as a shock absorber. Teeth have feelings. When you put ice on your skin it hurts. It's the same with teeth. Freezing temperatures affect their reactions. But do you know what really hurts their feelings? Not flossing. Too much sugar. Neglect.

Dentists don't just look at teeth, though. Within the mouth you also have gums, a tongue, cheeks and tonsils. It's a fascinating structure. Different kinds of dentists have different kinds of specialisms within the mouth. Some are experts at taking out teeth, while others do root canal and gum treatments. It's a specialism within a specialism, because as dentists we're already specialists within medicine. It's strange, because the mouth is treated as somewhat detached from the rest of the body. You go to the GP for your heart, your lungs, your kidneys, your spleen, your pancreas, but not your mouth. Your GP deals with everything but your mouth, which is a dentist's responsibility. I think it's time to put the mouth back into the body and think of dental and oral care as part of whole-body care!

It's a beautiful form of science. Dentistry has been my life for 22 years. I've come to know so many amazing people who have sat in my dental chair. Many of them with amazing teeth to match.

Plenty of my patients enjoy coming to get their teeth checked. They have full faith in me and are confident that they've looked after their mouth in the best possible way. They're the yin. But you know what comes with yin, don't you . . .

8

FEAR

Yang. Many, many people would rather 'give birth' or 'have full body tattoos' than go to the dentist. My friend has a great reply to the 'I'd rather give birth' comment; he just says, 'Whatever you want. You decide and then open wide.' I haven't built up the courage to try that one yet!!

Sometimes, I feel like I can't blame them. There are even times when *I* hate going to the dental practice, usually on a Monday morning!

We all have phobias – stuff we don't like and are afraid of without necessarily understanding why.

For me, it's the fear of heights. I'm not sure if it's an actual phobia, but I don't like being stuck up in the sky, hundreds of metres away from the ground. It freaks me out. And it's got worse over the years. I didn't used to have an issue with heights. You could have thrown me on a rollercoaster or flown me across the world and I wouldn't have batted an eyelid. Now, I can't help but wonder what would happen if we crashed. You won't see me on a rollercoaster any more. As you get older, you become more aware of your own mortality and all of the precious things in your life that you'd lose.

Other fears I've had for as long as I can remember. I've always had a dislike of certain creepy-crawlies. Worms? Not an issue. Woodlice? Absolutely fine. However, show me a big black house spider and I'll instinctively move away. It's just that they run around so fast that I find it unsettling. It's totally irrational. I know that the spider can't hurt me and that it's actually a helpful bug to have around but that doesn't make much difference.

One man's house spider is another man's dentist.

There's the petrifying prospect of the dental chair, the stranger in the tunic who sticks their fingers down your throat, the lack of control, the mouth full of wash, the gurgling, the gargling, the gagging, the hoovering, the drills, the needles forced into your gums, the potential to have teeth pulled out, the impending pain and the numbness that results in dribbling and the feeling that half your face is hanging off.

To those who have such fears, let me say one thing: dentists are *not bad people.*

That's right. We don't go home to our lair at the end of every working day to dream up more wicked ways to deprive the nation of their teeth.

We want you to have good teeth!

We want you to take pride in brushing.

And we want you to enjoy coming to the dentist.

Here's how . . .

The key to conquering fear is to find what you're afraid of and unlearn it. We are born with only two phobias: the fear of loud noises and the fear of falling. If you set off a firework next to a baby the loud bang is probably going to make them cry. If you trip them up or push them down the stairs, then not only are you a really horrible person who probably needs some help, but the fall you've put the baby through will also make them cry. Take that baby to the dentist and chances are they're not going to cry. If anything, they're going to be inquisitive. This is a chance to explore something new.

Any fear that isn't of falling or of loud noises has been learnt. It could have come from a bad experience. Maybe it stemmed from friends or family or from a film you've seen. If you've watched *Little Shop of*

Horrors or *The Dentist,* you'll know what I mean. In the former, Steve Martin plays a sadistic, nitrous oxide-addicted dentist, while in the latter, the psychotic protagonist pulls everyone's teeth out and then slashes their faces for good measure. Watch either film on a dark night and you're unlikely to be looking forward to your 8am check-up the next day.

You only need one influential person in your life to tell you that a visit to the dentist is painful for a phobia to start developing. If your parents are scared of going to the dentist and look apprehensive around their appointments, then chances are you will also adopt that fear. That's because you love and trust your parents – when you're younger, at least. What about hearing a horror story in the school playground? 'Oh my god, I went to the dentist the other day and it was so painful. He pulled out 12 of my teeth and made me sign my name in blood.' Wow. You wouldn't want to go to the dentist after hearing that.

We live in a culture where we love to talk about how terrible everything is. Good news doesn't sell papers. You might get the odd feel-good article on a Friday, but other than that it's an avalanche of doom, doom and more doom with a side portion of gloom. Why build something up when you can slag it off?

Which brings me to the touchy subject of reviews. These are so important to businesses these days. Restaurants and hotels invite guests to share their experiences on sites such as TripAdvisor. It's the same for dentists. Dental practices rely on good reviews to get more patients. The problem is that people are much more likely to tell the world about a bad experience than a good one. If a patient has 10 years' worth of efficient, pain-free appointments, then has one filling that hurts, what do you think they're going to remember? 'Oh my god, I had a filling that was so painful. Worst experience ever!'

Some people go to the dentist and actually do feel pain. They aren't made to sign their name in blood – at least not in my clinic – but some treatments can hurt a little. It was far worse 40 or 50 years ago. Back then, preventive dentistry wasn't a concept – or if it was, it equated to: take out all a patient's teeth and give them dentures by the age of 21. That was considered dentistry for the rich. Dentistry for the masses involved shoving a load of metal in the patient's mouth without so much as a 'how's your day?' Thank goodness dentistry has evolved, and rich people now want white teeth instead of no teeth. Although some choose a rather blinding shade of white – yes, I'm looking at you Mr Cowell . . . Big fan btw!

These days we look for early signs of problems in the mouth and try and stop them *before* they develop. Removing a tooth is the last resort rather than the solution. Typically, there's no pain involved in this process due to the progress in the most important drugs in medicine . . . anaesthetics!

Giving an anaesthetic injection can be a source of discomfort and it tends to be what patients are most afraid of: the needle. When they think of a needle, they picture a thick, 20-cm-long piece of metal with a sharp point that's hungry for their blood. The reality is far from this. The needles used in dentistry are really short and incredibly thin. Most of the time, patients don't even feel the needle pierce their skin. We can also apply a numbing gel to the patient's gum before an injection to make things even more comfortable.

In addition to a fear of pain, there's also a known condition called white coat hypertension. This isn't exclusive to dentistry. It also happens in other medical disciplines. The patient gets so worked up that their blood pressure increases – just because they're about to be examined. It can even happen before something as simple and painless as a check-up!

And then there's just the general fear of the unknown. Your dentist might not be good at communicating, and before you know it, you can be lying down in the chair, totally out of control and feeling vulnerable. And when the dentist's hand goes into your mouth, that only makes it worse.

When you visit your doctor, check-ups tend to be external. They might be looking at an outbreak of acne or a rash on your elbow. Even when they take blood, the doctor punctures your skin but it's still external. And, crucially, you can see what is happening – if you want to, anyway. But come to the dentist and most of the work is internal, and out of sight. The psychology is totally different. For some, it's terrifying. Especially when it comes to operations. Our anaesthetics only numb the pain. They don't knock you out, like they do when you have an operation in hospital. There's no 'one, two, three, goodnight Vienna' before waking up with the procedure long finished. Instead, you're awake the whole time. You hear the sound of the drill, the packing of the filling, all while not seeing what is going on in your mouth.

The most extreme solution for patients who fear their visits to the dentist is to simply stop going to have their teeth checked. The trouble with this approach is that the patient no longer has the benefit of preventative dentistry. Inevitably, things get worse. Teeth don't just fix themselves. Gum disease won't just go away. Dentistry is a science that requires intervention. And that doesn't mean trying it at home – I have seen many DIY dental disasters, from people pulling teeth with dirty pliers to using superglue to stick things back on! Believe me, that is not a good idea . . .

In many aspects of life, the longer you leave a problem, the more drastic the solution is likely to be. This is also true for dental problems; what's more the longer you leave it, the more costly it will be! Patients wait and wait, and when it finally erupts, chances are, they're not going to have a fabulous, pain-free experience at the dentist's. Their fear becomes a self-fulfilling prophecy.

It's down to dentists to change these attitudes around fear. An easy way to do this is to ensure people never learn fear in the first place. There's a campaign, Dental Check by One, that encourages parents to bring their children in for their first dental check-up before they turn one. It's all about normalising the process of going to the dentist.

When a baby comes in for their check-up, we

don't even look in their mouth. It's more about getting them into the environment and giving their parents some advice; providing them with some key dental tips and making sure everyone has a positive experience.

Another way to prevent fear is by educating our patients from an early age to look after their teeth. Ultimately, the best dentistry is no dentistry. Wouldn't it be amazing if your car servicing cost you £50 and the mechanic never found a problem? Imagine that no work ever needed to be done to your car. That'd be awesome. It never happens, though, because your car needs new tyres, an oil change, some new brakes – but that is normal because it drives around all sorts of environments. It encounters potholes, speed bumps, dirt tracks and, for those less skilled drivers, kerbs. It takes a lot of bashing and covers a lot of miles, meaning your mechanic often needs to do work on it. The same goes for your mouth. It's one of the most hostile areas in your body. It processes food multiple times a day, deals with all kinds of liquids, is used for talking, kissing, exchanging new bugs with old bugs. That's a lot of mouth mileage.

That's the message we want to get across to our patients, whatever their age! Normalise the visit, then normalise the process of looking after their mouth.

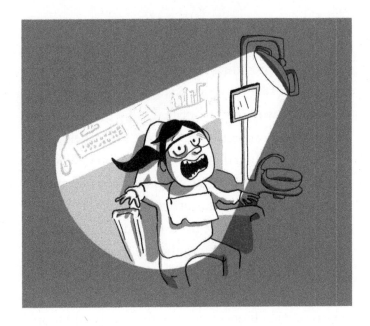

The better they look after it, the more miles it'll be able to do. Even better, they'll be less likely to need fillings, extensive gum treatment or teeth removed. And hopefully, that in turn will help prevent the development of a phobia of the dentist. Now, of course accidents can happen and if something goes wrong with the patient, we want them to know that we're there to help.

Certainly, it's never too late to unlearn a phobia. In extreme circumstances, there's always hypnosis. That was actually one of the modules on my dentistry course. Hypnosis can get people into the psychological state where they can unlearn fear, or at least put them into a relaxed mindset where they can deal with issues more easily. If it's the cost that horrifies them, you can hypnotise them to forget the fee!

For the most frightened patients, who just cannot unlearn their fear, dentists have to make procedures as bearable as possible, getting the job done quickly and with as much care and as little pain as they can manage. We can also use sedation to make patients more relaxed while they're having their treatments. They may never forget bad experiences they've had in the past, but with a bit of effort, they will never have bad experiences again. All the time, a dentist can reassure them. They can tell them of the scientific advances, the better materials and the more sophisticated treatments. Take fluoride, for example. This naturally occurring mineral is present in all water supplies in varying amounts. It helps protect the teeth and prevents the bacteria that causes tooth decay. Often, the level isn't high enough to give these benefits, so there are community water fluoridation schemes that increase the amount of fluoride to a level that can be beneficial.

In the US, fluoride has been added to water supplies

since the mid-1940s and I feel this has helped Americans to have stronger teeth.

The ultimate way to prevent fear, however, isn't only down to the dentist. It's down to the patient to make sure they take good care of their pegs.

9

MYTH BUSTERS

While we're on the subject of looking after the treasure trove that is your mouth, I thought I'd take the chance to bust some of the Loch Ness Monster-sized myths about dentistry that are out there. Rumours become whispers, which become hushed opinions, which eventually find their way to becoming 'facts', much to the distress of dentists and other medical professionals.

Remember when your mum told you that eating carrots would make you see in the dark? How about when she told you that if you swallowed chewing gum it would stay in your stomach for seven years? Yep, that's the kind of stuff I'm getting at.

Not to worry: this chapter is going to demolish the most popular myths in dentistry. No longer will you be misled in the era of fake news. So here goes . . .

Myth #1

Only refined sugars found in products such as sweets, chocolates and fizzy drinks damage your teeth. Naturally occurring sugars, such as those in fruit, are fine.

False!

While refined sugars are worse for your teeth, eating any type excessively will cause cavities. Factor in that fruits also contain acids that can erode the enamel of the tooth and you start to see that everything isn't rosy. Now, I wouldn't tell anyone to never eat fruit as the vitamins and other goodness within them are beneficial. It's just something to be mindful of – consuming it in moderation is fine. Also, beware of dried fruit: not only is it essentially concentrated sugar, but it's extremely sticky too, meaning it clings to your teeth. To limit the negative impact on your teeth, eat something alkaline like cheese afterwards to help neutralise the pH of your mouth. And keep sugary drinks to mealtimes, ideally diluting them with ice and drinking them through a straw. Oh yeah, and fresh fruit juices are also a problem . . . when you blend fruits, you release the sugars from the fibres and essentially create a really sugary drink. Plus you often

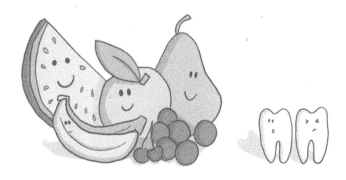

made up of loads more fruit than you would actually eat in one sitting! For example it takes three oranges to make your average glass of orange juice. Sorry to bust the juicing bubble . . .

Myth #2
If your gums bleed when you brush them, stop brushing as it may damage them further.

False!
Bleeding gums is a sign that there's some inflammation in your gums, probably due to a build-up of plaque

and debris. Brushing will help to remove this build-up and hopefully calm the inflammation. If it doesn't, then get yourself off to the dentist for a proper assessment. But of course, you remembered that from the last chapter . . . I hope . . .

Myth #3
Bad breath is always a sign of poor oral health.

False!
Of course, tooth decay and gum disease are both causes of halitosis or bad breath, but they are far from being the only cause.

The smell could be caused by bacteria on the tongue – that great big flappy thing in your mouth harbours loads of them. It's grooved, lumpy, bumpy and furry. The bacteria love it there. They set up camp, get their mates round and make a right mess. They let off some sulphurm compounds that smell like rotten eggs – not at all pleasant! And bacteria aren't the only things on your tongue. Stick it out and you may be able to see some white slough, which is essentially a collection of dead cells, food and gunk. 'What can I do?' I hear you cry.

Scrape your tongue dude!!!

Dentistry has evolved so far that we now have dedicated tongue brushes and tongue scrapers. Start using one. Your other half will certainly thank you for it.

Bad breath could also be due to inadequate flow of saliva into the mouth. Stay hydrated, and if you notice your mouth is continually or constantly dry, speak with your doctor or dentist. It could be due to an underlying condition or a medication you are taking.

Another cause of bad breath could be stomach problems. The gases from your gut can actually come up and out through your mouth, making your breathe smell. It is worth ruling this out too.

Finally, a personal favourite of mine: the smell could be due to tonsilloliths. What's a tonsillolith? I hear you cry. Well . . . they are tonsil stones; a hard, white, crusty build-up of bacteria, dead cells and debris that get stuck in the nooks and crannies of your tonsils and they absolutely stink! You may be able to see them – they look like grains of rice – and they can often be coughed out. If you persistently get them, the only real treatment is to have the tonsils removed, so having an appointment with an ear, nose and throat doctor would be something to consider.

Myth #4
You don't need to brush baby teeth as they fall out anyway.

False!
Children don't lose their last baby teeth until around the age of 12. If you don't keep those baby teeth healthy until they fall out, then you're going to have problems. Cavities in baby teeth can worsen quickly and cause pain, as well as infections – and no one wants to see their little one suffering. Also, early loss of baby teeth due to infections can delay or interrupt the eruption of the adult teeth, so it is vital to keep them healthy.

It's best to start brushing your baby's teeth as soon as they appear. Use age-appropriate toothpaste to ensure that they have the right levels of fluoride and keep watch so they don't swallow it. You will need to teach children to spit – doing a demo can help. I used to brush my children's teeth at bath times so they could dribble and make as much mess as they wanted.

Myth #5
You should brush your teeth immediately after eating.

False!

Bacteria in your mouth eat the food that you feed them. The acid by-product they release weakens the enamel of the teeth. And brushing immediately after eating will only rub this acid into the teeth, weakening the enamel further. Let the saliva do its thing in neutralising the pH of the mouth and wait at least 30 minutes after eating before you brush.

Myth #6

A cup of milk before bed will give you strong, healthy teeth.

False!

Milk contains calcium, so drinking it can be beneficial for teeth. However, it also contains the natural sugar lactose, which can weaken enamel over time if you drink it before bed and don't brush afterwards. If you want a drink last thing before bed, choose water.

Myth #7

Brush firmly to give your mouth the best clean.

False!

Teeth are hard, gums are not. If you brush too hard, it can wear away the gum and cause gum recession. Instead, use either a medium- or soft-bristled manual brush, pressing gently while you do a circular motion at 45 degrees to the gums or an electric toothbrush, keeping it still, getting the right angle and guiding it along the teeth for maximum effect. Massage, don't force!

Myth #8
Braces are for teenagers.

False!
You're never too old for braces. Teeth can always be moved, and if they're particularly wonky, you could reduce the chances of gum disease and tooth decay occurring by doing so. Also, the cosmetic aspect of having straight teeth is something to consider.

Myth #9
Rinse your mouth – with water or mouthwash – after brushing.

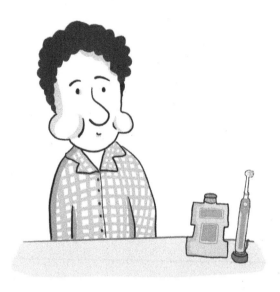

False!

Rinsing washes off the fluoride and all the other good mineral ingredients in your toothpaste. Spit, don't rinse, and make sure those minerals work their magic on your teeth. If you're going to use mouthwash, do so at a different time from brushing. Note that it should be an adjunct to effective manual cleaning, not a replacement for brushing and flossing. For those who are more prone to gum disease or have sensitive teeth, specific mouthwashes can be very useful and there are even some dedicated to combating bad breath, but in general, I like to think of mouthwash like wax on a car. Putting wax on a dirty car isn't going to do much good. You need to clean your car thoroughly before you get the wax involved. Only then can it do what it's supposed to and add protection.

Myth #10
You only need to floss when you have food stuck in your teeth.

False!
A tooth is a 3D structure. When you clean the front, you're only cleaning part of that structure. The same goes for the back. Where you really earn your dental health gold star is by brushing in the pockets between the tooth and gum. These 1–2mm gaps under your gum are bacteria's favourite place to grow. They form a large colony of sticky biofilm called plaque, and without effective cleaning, this plaque will harden and form tartar, which clings to the teeth and cannot be removed without the help of a dental professional.

Brushing at a 45-degree angle to the tooth helps to clean the pocket out, but to really get deep into the crevice, you need to do some interdental cleaning, by using either an interdental brush or floss. There are many implements for this: interdental brushes (they look like tiny bog-brushes), floss-picks (floss in a handle, looks like a catapult), special toothpicks (not a fan of wooden ones, though, as they can cause more damage than good) and interdental irrigators that shoot water into the gaps between the teeth. Which one you use can depend on several factors: the size of the gaps between your teeth, how crowded or squished your teeth are and also your manual dexterity, which plays a huge part. Using floss or even interdental brushes can be very fiddly, which is why we often see patients give it a go but then stop as it feels like a chore. Ask your dentist or hygienist and to recommend the tools that will best suit your mouth and teeth, and then it's just a case of doing it regularly as part of your daily routine.

Myth #11
Any teeth can be whitened.

False!
Lots of over-the-counter products claim that they can whiten your teeth. To be fair, some can make the teeth appear 'whiter', but that is because they are removing external staining. To get true colour change, you need

to deal with the internal colour, which can only be done by visiting your dentist.

The first thing dentists will do is check that your teeth are suitable for whitening. We will have to make sure that there is no evidence of gum disease or tooth decay, cavities or infections and that you've proved you can look after your teeth. To look at cosmetic treatments without first ensuring teeth are healthy is a huge mistake, which is why a lot of people come unstuck when they get teeth whitening done by anyone other than a dental professional.

After your dentist has assessed your teeth, they can recommend home whitening or in-surgery whitening and give you instructions on how to do this. The best results always come from combining your teeth whitening with these four key principles:

- Brush twice a day
- Reduce sugar intake
- See your dentist at regular intervals
- Clean inbetween your teeth with floss or interdental brushes

Repeat.

And don't let anyone tell you otherwise.

Myth #12
Oral cancer is a disease of the elderly.

False!

Anyone can be affected by oral cancer – whether they have teeth or not. Though it is most common in men over the age of 40, oral cancer is becoming more common in younger patients. It can appear anywhere in the mouth, on the tongue or lips. It often appears as a painless ulcer that doesn't heal by itself after a week or two, or as white or red patches.

But it can be hard to detect early cancer lesions because they don't cause pain or symptoms. So, who's going to spot it? Dentists!!! Which is why regular check-ups are essential, even if you have no teeth!

The main causes of oral cancer are tobacco and alcohol – especially when they're used together. Overexposure to sunlight is a contributor and can affect the lower lip in particular. Using a sunblock on the lips can help prevent this. Research has also linked the human papillomavirus (HPV) to oral cancer. HPV can be spread through oral sex, so necessary precautions should always be taken.

All cancers are bad, and oral cancer is a particularly bad one, not least because the mouth is close to the lymph nodes in the neck, so the cancer can spread quickly to the rest of the body. If you visit your dentist regularly, they will be able to identify sinister lesions at the earliest point. If left late, the treatment is very invasive and has a much worse long-term prognosis.

Treatment almost always involves cutting out any area that's affected – which could include parts of the tongue, jaw, face or neck, and this can have major impacts on quality-of-life post-op. Early detection is key and may result in a much easier treatment modality and much better long-term survival.

10

A WORLD WITHOUT DENTISTS
(WELL, ALMOST)

When coronavirus hit in March 2020, the dental industry ground to a halt. All of a sudden, we could no longer see patients and there was uncertainty everywhere. There was also a lot of frustration. After all, in dentistry we've been dealing with transmissible diseases forever. Dentists have always worn masks. We've always worn gloves. Visors have always been there. Wiping equipment down after every patient is and always has been standard practice. Dental clinics already had in-house sterilisation.

If there was one industry that should have been unaffected by Covid, it was dentistry.

In fact, a dental clinic was probably one of the cleanest places you could have gone. And that's with us being inside your mouth and standing only around 20 cm away from you!

The government didn't think so. They shut us all down until more research had been done. Fair enough, but that wasn't the case in many other countries.

So instead of still seeing my wonderful patients in the flesh, my team and I had to speak to them over the phone. In case you hadn't guessed, the phone isn't the most effective method of diagnosing someone's dental concerns. As dentists, we need to be in their mouth, assessing them, treating them.

For weeks, then months, I'd finish a day of work with my ear aching from having it pressed to a phone for hours and having it bashed by patients. Then, an announcement from the government. 'Great!' we thought. How wrong we were . . . The government would now allow us to see patients, but only if it was an emergency. And only if they absolutely had to come in.

The changes that were then proposed to allow us to deal with these patients would make our jobs even more difficult. Worse, there was no real evidence for them.

The most crippling was the concept of a 'fallow period'. This arose from the theory that if you are working on a patient who has Covid and are doing an AGP – an aerosol generating procedure, such as drilling – inside their mouth, it may potentially spray Covid droplets around the room. These droplets then take an hour to settle, after which time, they are wiped and cleaned. If this isn't done, they can potentially transmit Covid to others who come into contact with them. Under the new guidelines, then, we'd have to wait a full hour between seeing patients. Even then, we'd only be allowed to wipe down surfaces after the hour had passed, so in reality it was slightly more. What was once an eight-hour day in which you'd see

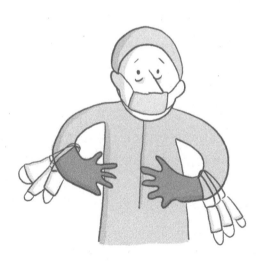

30 or so patients had become an eight-hour day in which you could see seven patients; eight if you didn't bother with lunch, cleaned like Speedy Gonzales and went some way beyond the nine-to-five.

Thirty patients a day down to seven? It felt impossible to run a business.

The money coming in took a hit. And the money going out took a big Muhammad Ali uppercut to the face.

Nobody really knew what PPE was before the pandemic. They were more likely to think that PPE was what you had to study if you wanted to become prime minister. That worked for us dentists because it kept PPE costs nice and low. We could get a box of gloves for £2.50, for example. Fast forward a couple of months and that same box became £22.

£22!

Bruv . . .

You use the gloves once and then chuck them away. So you need more gloves, which cost more £22s.

And it wasn't just gloves I was wearing. I was pretty much having to walk around looking like a kebab shop owner with my apron on.

'Hello sir, would you like chilli sauce or garlic sauce?' I'd ask my confused patients upon arrival.

'Why are you wearing a hazmat suit?' they'd respond.

We'd have our back-and-forth and then the appointment would be over and everything would be thrown in the bin. Even if I wore a washable gown, the amount of plastics that ended up in our bin was no joke. We're out here trying to save the world but in the dental industry we are now fighting a losing battle. Paper gowns aren't an option. They don't like getting wet. With much of PPE, plastic is the only solution. Poor Greta would have a heart attack if she saw the contents of my bin each day.

Not only were the day-to-day costs rising, but we also had to invest in air purifying systems, as the government said that they could only relax their fallow period rules as long as we used them. Basically, these units replace the air every 10 minutes, meaning that the fallow period could be brought down from an hour to 10 minutes. But this came at a cost – £2000 for each air purifyer, which was a hefty outlay! We all wanted to get back to seeing more patients so we had to fork out the money. I bought three . . . Lovely. With all the added extras, what was previously a difficult job had become a very difficult job.

Finally, we were allowed to see our check-up

patients again. In some ways, it felt like the light at the end of the tunnel. For so long we'd just been triaging and dealing with a handful of patients who required urgent care. But in other ways, it felt like we were about to enter the biggest, darkest tunnel that dentistry has ever seen.

Not seeing check-up patients for a year meant that there was one year's worth of backlog. That backlog had to be fitted into a diary where there were also plenty of emergencies. Never had we been busier. The phone seemed to be ringing non-stop with people asking to be registered as an NHS patient. Lockdown had made them reassess their lives and maybe made them realise that it had been a long time since their last check-up. That brought up another problem: we were unable to take on new NHS patients because my NHS associate dentists had a massive backlog of existing patients.

However, my private associate dentists were able to take on private patients. The way Covid had decimated the industry, private patients gave a lifeline to many clinics and there seemed to be more private patients than ever before. We put that down to the 'Zoom Boom'.

The Zoom Boom theory suggests that because

much of the population was stuck indoors during the lockdowns and spending all day working from home, they saved quite a bit of money. They didn't go away on holiday, didn't go for that Saturday morning coffee, didn't go out for dinner. Yet throughout that time, they were receiving their salary as normal. On their video calls, they spent a lot of time staring at themselves on camera – far more than normal. Over time, what once seemed normal began to be seen as an imperfection. 'Wow,' it got people thinking, 'maybe I should do something about my hair/face/skin/nose/teeth.'

As soon as clinics opened again for non-emergency procedures, teeth jobs became a big thing.

Clinics got busier with cosmetic treatments. They're life-changing for the patient, and also enjoyable for the dentist. Nobody thanks you when you do root canal on them, but they love you when you make their teeth whiter. That made private treatment more attractive for lots of dentists. And it isn't the only reason why more clinics are turning to private treatment.

With the NHS, the pricing scheme is structured in bands of treatment, and what you pay as a patient remains the same regardless of the volume of treatment. Let's take a filling, for example. Go private and it'll cost you around £150, depending on the size.

On the NHS, the same treatment would be Band 2, which is £65.20. However, within Band 2 you would also be entitled to a check-up, X-rays, a scale and polish, and any number of fillings, root canals and extractions that are clinically necessary. All for the same fee of £65.20.

Let's use an analogy . . .

If you go to the pub and you pay £5 for a pint, fine. That's cool for all involved. But if you then go to another pub and pay £5 for an unlimited number of pints, that's not so cool. You might have one mad night followed by one humongous hangover, but pretty soon that pub landlord is going to go bust and there'll be no more pub. Where are you going to get your pints from when that happens?

That, in a nutshell, is the problem with NHS dentistry.

A small filling takes 30 minutes. Thirty fillings, however, require four hours every week for quite a number of weeks. Dentists have to give up all that time for £63.80. It'd actually be more cost efficient for them to pay the patient to go elsewhere! Especially if they have a big waiting list of Zoom Boom patients.

Who suffers most as a result of this? The people who need those NHS clinics most desperately. Those

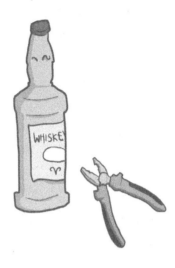

who have lots of money will be fine. They can afford to go private. Yet for those who haven't been to the dentist in a long time, who are already struggling with money, it becomes impossible to get treatment if they suddenly get problems. No clinic will be able to afford to take them on, and so those people will be the ones who have to resort to DIY dentistry. Think supergluing your teeth back into your gums, or trying to pull teeth out with a spanner and a bottle of whiskey. It's those people who will end up with mouth cancer that goes undetected.

Many dental clinics have a mix of NHS and private services. Those that were purely private took a big hit during Covid. Those that were purely NHS kept their funding, while the rest sat in the middle. The way that NHS dental funding works is that you receive an exact amount of money to provide an exact number of Units of Dental Activity (UDAs). To give you an idea, a check-up, X-rays and a scale and polish gives the clinic one UDA, whereas a Band 2, which I talked about earlier, gives the clinic three UDAs.

Very early on in the pandemic, the NHS clocked that clinics weren't going to hit their UDA targets. They adapted the requirements, so that as long as you were triaging patients was fine: they'd still pay 100% of the money. In my clinic, that commitment allowed me to pay my staff, my bills and to keep the clinic open. Private clinics, where there were no NHS treatments, got nothing. All they could do was furlough staff and hope they could ride the storm while still paying their rents and their bills.

Talk about creating more friction between state and private!

'I can't believe these NHS dentists are getting all this money!' the private dentists moaned.

'Well we're the ones who have been seeing 30 plus patients a day for the last 20 years while you've been living it up,' the NHS dentists retorted.

With the funding from the NHS and the reduction in UDA, however, NHS dentists were finally getting to experience what private dentistry could be like. There was still plenty of work to be getting on with, but they no longer had to cram appointments into every nook and cranny of the day. And they liked it.

So when the pandemic eased and the NHS asked clinics to do 20% of their usual target, that was still fine. NHS dentists were seeing 12 patients a day, going out of the room between patients and writing up their notes, doing their referrals, catching up on bits and bobs. They were no longer running late all the time, nor having to stay late.

Then 20% went up to 40%. Then to 60%. 65%. 85%.

Just as the work ramped up, the Omicron wave of Covid arrived. People were dropping left, right and centre. Patients cancelled last minute. Staff were unable to work. People had to isolate. Suddenly, those same dentists who had adapted nicely to their new life of 20% of their usual work with 100% of the money were under a lot of pressure – just as they'd been easing back into their profession.

'How am I ever going to meet 85% of my targets?' dentists wailed. No matter how much they were reminded that they used to meet 100% of their targets, it didn't help. The pandemic has changed so many people's mindsets and dentists are no exception. The days of smashing through 30 patients a day without coming up for air are finished. That's for the better.

The NHS now wants us all to get back to normal but because of Covid, there is no normal. The pandemic has had a huge impact on the number of practising dentists. Many NHS dentists became accustomed to fewer patients and better hours, so they switched to private dentistry. Some NHS dentists have reduced their number of clinical days and some have sadly stepped away from the industry all together. Overseas dentists, whom we relied upon heavily in the past, haven't been able to come over for their conversion courses because of Covid. Many had already left because of Brexit. Graduates don't want to start off in the NHS because they don't want to bang out units of activity, even though that's the way dentistry has always been done.

I've been advertising for an associate at my clinic for more than two months and yet nobody wants to do it. I'm supposed to be The Singing Dentist, bruv! If I'm struggling to get someone in, imagine what it's like for other clinics. (If you're reading this and that sounds like the job for you, by the way, there's an application form in the back of the book.)

Ultimately, we need reform. The NHS contract in its current condition was introduced in 2006. In 2009, the government announced they were going to start pilot schemes to improve dentistry in the country. They realised what they were doing wasn't fit for purpose. However, more than a decade later nothing has changed. Every dentist wants to care for each individual patient. We want to take pride in our dentistry. We just need a system in which we can do that properly.

We find ourselves in a place of uncertainty. I want to remain positive and hopeful that, because the pandemic highlighted all the flaws in the system, it will change for the better. Yet at the same time, I fear nothing will improve because it hasn't for so long. I fear that the Great Resignation will become the Even Greater Resignation and that fewer and fewer people will be able to access quality dentistry.

No matter what happens, one thing that I am certain of is that dentists will always hold their duty of care in the highest regard. Even if it comes at the expense of their business, or their own mental or physical health, dentists will put their patients first. They'll continue to help patients look and feel good. And hopefully, with every treatment, they can help to change the perception of dentistry, one check-up at a time!

11

WHY I SING

Opportunities can come from the strangest of places. When you're a dentist, that can include the dental chair itself. A dentist colleague had a patient in for a routine check-up on a routine day in a routine week. During the small talk, he discovered that the patient in his chair worked in artists and repetoire (A&R) for a record label.

'Have you heard of The Singing Dentist?' he asked.

'Hmm,' the patient mused. 'I think so but I'm not sure. Is that the guy who sings about sausage rolls?'

After the check-up, the A&R representative went home and typed my name into YouTube. He checked out one of my videos, then a second. Then a third. It turned out that he loved them. He couldn't stop laughing and was convinced that I needed to do a proper song.

So, he sent me a message.

When the email landed in my inbox, I tried my best not to get excited. Having flirted with record deals in the past without anything crazy ever materialising, I'd learnt not to get carried away. There was a kind of tingle going through my body, though. *I can't get excited by this yet, but it might lead to something exciting.*

The emails flew back and forth and plans were made. Soon, the wheels were in motion and the tingles were getting more intense. I suggested we use 'I Like Your Molars Molars'. I'd already released it as a parody and the song resonates with a wide demographic. There are those who first heard the Reel 2 Real classic when it was released in 1993. Then there is the younger generation who were introduced to it in the 2005 'Madagascar' version. The 434,000 views it had garnered on my YouTube channel proved its potential. The record label agreed with me that we should use 'I Like Your Molars Molars' and suggested we bring it out as a Christmas single.

So I set about re-recording it.

I had first thought of the parody after my kids had watched *Madagascar*. They were going wild around the house as usual, both singing 'I like to move it, move

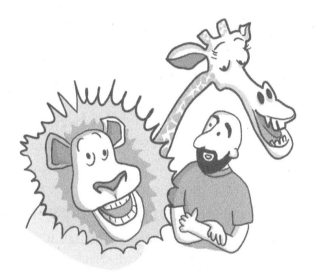

it' at the top of their lungs. 'Hold on,' I thought. 'I can do something here.' The changes to the lyrics came seamlessly.

All patients over the world
Original Singing Dentist 'pun your case, man
I loooooove when my patients keep their recalls
Cah when you don't miss appointments
I can keep your teeth nice and clean and healthy

I belted out the lyrics once again. Recreated, re-recorded and remastered for an actual proper record label! When the record label sent the tune back to me after they'd worked their magic I was blown away. It sounded amazing!

We opted against releasing it in time for Christmas. I'd heard that LADBaby was going for his second consecutive Christmas number one and we decided to delay the release. LADBaby's sausage-roll-inspired parodies are amazing! We all agreed that summer would be the best time for the song. It was fun and bubbly, the perfect anthem for those long, never-ending days of sun. But then coronavirus hit. Hold on . . . wouldn't it be amazing to release the single and donate all the profits to NHS charities? That way I'd be helping with both my dentistry and my music. My management team was happy with that, the record label was happy with that and so we did exactly that.

The evening before the song was officially released, I sat in my office staring at my computer screen. The page was open on iTunes and there it was. My official single produced by a proper record label available for pre-order. It had finally happened. I carried on staring. I never wanted to look away.

The reaction when it was officially released was incredible. Receiving messages from people I didn't know saying how much they loved the song and how their children were playing it 30 times a day gave me such a buzz.

Not everything was plain sailing. Being in lockdown made it hard to promote the single. Whereas LADBaby had gone out into the streets with a megaphone and shouted at randomers to buy his record, I had to do everything from the safety of my own home. Interviews and PR opportunities had to be done virtually. Even the music video had to be filmed from my house! I bought a green screen cloth off the internet, hung it in my office and filmed myself dancing in front of it. A friend of mine then helped to edit it and voilà: my first official music video for my first official record!

And I didn't want to stop there. My parody songs have continued to garner millions of views from all around the world. Influencers and celebrities have watched and loved my videos and opened me up to new demographics. I'd love music to be part of everything that I do moving forward. While my work as The Singing Dentist has me singing about teeth, I'd also like to break out of my niche and pursue other musical projects (don't worry, I'll still be active as The Singing Dentist!).

And I hope I'll always keep the DJing up. During lockdown I livestreamed myself on the decks at the self-styled Club Conservatoire (not quite as posh as it sounds). I'd love to be like Idris Elba, who also has a passion for DJing. While he's not acting, you can sometimes catch him doing a set in Ibiza. I'm not saying that I'm on Idris Elba's level, but when you have a passion for something and get an opportunity to do it, it's very exciting and rewarding. When it's a passion, it isn't about the money. I don't necessarily want to go on tour and have a sold-out show in Vegas (unless any readers out there want me to, then I'm down!). I just love music.

I've never really had a plan in place for what I want to achieve. It's more a case of going with the flow. I keep on doing what I'm doing, keep on being me. That authenticity is key. My platform has allowed me to work with businesses, set up my own creating my own dental products and do plenty of media work. Exploring the comedy element also interests me. People seem to think I'm funny and I know that I've got a funny face. EYEBROWS, anyone? Comedy acting would be great. Maybe presenting would be fun. The dream would have to be my own radio show where I could pick the music

I played and interview a whole load of people in the music business.

I'd love to use my platform as The Singing Dentist to help educate people around dentistry. I want to remove the stigma, to stop people thinking that dental practices are horrible places where you go to get tortured by dentists who make loads of money by hurting you. I want more people to start loving their dentist! Part of it is education, but part of it is also about improving the dental experience. Dental clinics should be seen more as a health service, much in the way that spas are. Think about it: nobody hates going to the spa even though a massage can hurt. Having a facial with specific peels can definitely hurt. The same goes for having liposuction or laser work done. But because it's the spa and it's health focused people look forward to their visit. We need to make dentistry have the same vibe, to play up a dental practice's role as a health service, to make it more luxurious.

That education and changing of attitudes begins with my patients. All the experiences I've had over recent years have had an incredible effect on me, but my patients help to keep me grounded. They won't let me get carried away – I'm still Jenny from the block!

They may say they've seen me on the telly or that their friend shared my video on their social media channel, but at the end of the day they'll ask me to look inside their mouth. They've come to understand I have commitments other than dentistry and the vast majority don't complain if I ever have to cancel their appointments because an urgent media opportunity has come up. All of my Singing Dentist work has helped to attract new patients and build even stronger ties with my existing patients. Some laugh when they see me and say, 'What are you still doing here? I expected you to be in Hollywood by now.' They reckon I'll drop dentistry and take up acting any second. AND THEY'RE ABSOLUTELY RIGHT, I'D DROP IT IN A HEARTBEAT! No, I'm joking.

The main reason that I'll always be involved in dentistry is the patients. They make me laugh, smile and cry. They share their deepest hopes and fears with me. And those experiences we share have a big impact on my working life.

Patient Y was 25 years old when she came through the door of my dental practice. It was her first time setting foot inside a dental clinic. Her teeth had never been professionally checked.

Her mum accompanied her. It was her mum who

spoke to the receptionist, her mum who booked the appointment and her mum who greeted me.

'Hello,' she said. 'This is Patient Y. She doesn't talk.'

Patient Y looked at me, totally silent.

'OK, that's fine, have a seat.' I guided her into the dental chair and asked her to open her mouth.

'She's got a bit of pain here and a bit more pain there,' her mum told me, pointing at the affected areas.

I could tell she needed some work doing, which was understandable, as she had never seen a dentist before. Some teeth needed to be taken out, others filled and one needed root canal treatment. Her teeth and gums also needed a deep clean.

With a case like this, building rapport and trust is imperative and you can't just dive in and start injecting, drilling and hacking away. You have to build things up slowly and develop a trusting relationship. Patient Y had first decided to come for an appointment because she was a fan of the Singing Dentist videos I put out on YouTube. That helped me earn her trust, so I had to be very mindful I didn't take that trust for granted.

The first appointment was just a check-up and we managed a tiny bit of cleaning. We got her booked in again and a few weeks later she returned with her mum.

Again, she was totally silent while her mum did all the talking.

This time I gave her a small filling. There was no reaction. The filling hadn't been an issue and she coped amazingly well, so at the next appointment we went to the next stage, then the next stage, then the next stage. Eventually, we got to the point where I carried out her root canal treatment.

Still, she remained silent, her mum doing the talking.

At the end of the session, her mum told me that Patient Y would love to buy one of my Singing Dentist T-shirts. A few weeks before, I had received a small shipment that I planned to give out for promotion. They came in grey, white and blue and I'd worn them in a Facebook Live post I'd made.

'They're not really for sale,' I told Patient Y's mum. 'But you can have one, it's not a problem. Which colour would you like?'

Patient Y looked up at me. Out of the corner of her mouth, quietly, so quietly, she said 'grey.'

There was a moment of shock, her mum was aghast and actually burst into tears.

'Oh my god, she's talking! She's talking! She's never spoken to anyone outside of our house!'

'What size are you?' I asked, giving her my full attention.

'Medium,' Patient Y replied, a little louder this time.

At our next appointment, I went about my work as usual and at the end, as she hopped out of the chair, Patient Y said, 'Thank you.' Again, her mum became emotional – we could all see this was a big milestone for the family.

At the next appointment a few weeks later, Patient Y's mum was nowhere to be seen. Patient Y had decided to come in all by herself.

'Hello, how are you?' she asked, clambering into the chair. She started chatting away like many of my patients do, and since then she hasn't stopped. We had now started to fit some clear braces for her, at her request, to realign her teeth and straighten them. I saw her every three weeks for nine months. The transformation was incredible. In the teeth, obviously, but more so in her! Such confidence, such courage. She genuinely seemed like a different person.

Having built up such a great relationship with her, I asked her if I could tell her story in this book.

Thankfully, she accepted and was even happy to share her side of it. So, I'd like to introduce Patient Y . . . Lucy.

'Hello, my name is Lucy and I'm 30 years old. I'm from Basingstoke and I am delighted to be a patient of The Singing Dentist.

'I had never been to a dentist before due to having selective mutism, which means I cannot talk in certain situations and I have social anxiety. This has caused me to be extremely fearful of visiting the dentist and I lack confidence in meeting people.

'I came across the Singing Dentist parodies on social media and loved them. The parodies were great – fun and also informative at the same time. After researching him and finding out that his dental practice was close by, I decided I wanted to go to that dentist. He came across as someone who genuinely loves his job and cares for his patients. This was a dentist that I felt confident enough to go to.

'I attended the first few visits with my mum. I enjoyed the experience because he made me feel calm and not nervous at all. Although I did not say a word to him until a couple of visits later, he was very welcoming. My friends and family can't believe that I actually enjoy visiting the dentist and that it is something I always look forward to. During my time there, I love hearing what the next parody will be or what TV show he's on next.

'I was able to start talking to Milad and gained more confidence as time went on and now am able to go there by myself, which was something I could not do before. I have been a patient of his since 2017 and my teeth look so much better now, which has given me so much confidence in smiling and talking to people.

'Without stumbling across the Singing Dentist, I would never have gone to the dentist to get my teeth seen to. Milad is genuinely one of the nicest people I've met, he's a great dentist, very supportive and fun to be around.'

If you're reading this now, Lucy, thank you for being a great patient!

You see, we dentists aren't all bad!!

ACKNOWLEDGEMENTS

Writing a book is something I've always wanted to do and I was super excited to be given the opportunity. However, I soon found out that this is far from a solitary process. I would like to thank everyone who has backed me from the start. I am deeply grateful to the many friends and family members who have supported me throughout this journey. Your encouragement, feedback, and unwavering belief has helped me to stay to focused and motivated.

First and foremost, I would like to thank my wife Joanne, for her unending support and understanding. Your patience and willingness to listen to my voice notes, scribblings and musings made this book possible. To my kids, I'd like to say, daddy loves you and hopefully you'll read this one day.

To my parents, thank you for always believing in me and supporting my dreams, no matter how crazy they may seem. Your love and encouragement continue to spur me on in all I do. And to my extended family, thank you for your support. Your belief in me and my abilities means the world to me.

To my dear friends, you know who you are. Thank you for cheering me on and always being there to chat when I need it.

To my dental colleagues, thank you for your insights and suggestions, they have helped me to shape this book into the best it could be.

To Seth, thank you for all you have done. Without your skills, this book wouldn't be what it is. Thanks for listening to my chats and helping to turn them into actual words.

And finally, a massive thank you to all my followers and supporters. Without all of you, I wouldn't be doing what I'm doing and I'm eternally grateful for your love over all these years. The comments and encouragement I get from you makes all the hard work worthwhile and this book would not have been possible without you.

I hope you all enjoy reading it as much as I have enjoyed writing it.

ABOUT THE AUTHOR

Dr Milad Shadrooh is a dentist and owner of Chequers Dental Surgery in Basingstoke. Outside of dentistry, Milad hit the headlines as the The Singing Dentist, with his educational and entertaining dental parody songs gaining a total of over 250 million views so far. Milad is the go-to media dental clinician with appearances on ITV's *This Morning*, *Good Morning Britain* and *Lorraine*, BBC News, Sky News and countless radio programmes. He's been voted the 'Most Influential Person' in Dentistry three times in the last four years.